The Dean Vaughn
Total Retention System™

MEDICAL TERMINOLOGY
350

Second Edition

Learning Guide

Produced and Published by
DCM/INSTRUCTIONAL SYSTEMS

ISBN 0-914901-12-5

DCM/Product number 15028-2

Printed in the United States of America

This Learning Guide will interact with all previously dated audio-visual program presentations of the Dean Vaughn Learning System Applied to Medical Terminology.

Ninth Printing, 2008

DCM/INSTRUCTIONAL SYSTEMS, a division of DCM Systems Incorporated   P.O. Box 96   Westwood, MA 02090

Table of Contents

† Previous Edition Substitution Page(s) included

▬▬ MEDICAL TERMINOLOGY 350 ▬▬

Pretest

Name_____ Date_____

Number Correct:	_____
Possible Score:	350
Percent Correct:	_____ %

☞ **Important**:

Clearly print the meaning of each element in the blank where indicated. If you do not know the meaning, leave the blank empty and move on to the next element.

Please do not feel uncomfortable taking this pretest. You are not expected to know the meanings at this time. The purpose of this exercise is only to establish a basis for measuring your accomplishment upon completing the program.

Element	Meaning	Element	Meaning
1. gastr-	_____	26. -algia	_____
2. cardi-	_____	27. crani-	_____
3. megal-	_____	28. end-	_____
4. -itis	_____	29. hemi-	_____
5. dermat-	_____	30. -oid	_____
6. plast-	_____	31. hyper-	_____
7. cerebr-	_____	32. cyst-	_____
8. path-	_____	33. chole-	_____
9. -ectomy	_____	34. hypo-	_____
10. enter-	_____	35. -scop-	_____
11. -osis	_____	36. hyster-	_____
12. -otomy	_____	37. -ostomy	_____
13. aden-	_____	38. para-	_____
14. angi-	_____	39. -lysis	_____
15. -oma	_____	40. cervic-	_____
16. nephr-	_____	41. chondr-	_____
17. hepat-	_____	42. cyan-	_____
18. arthr-	_____	43. hem(at)-	_____
19. blephar-	_____	44. ost-	_____
20. -ologist	_____	45. psycho-	_____
21. rhin-	_____	46. lip-	_____
22. gingiv-	_____	47. my-	_____
23. -malacia	_____	48. lith-	_____
24. -ology	_____	49. ophthalm- opt-	_____
25. spasm	_____	50. proct-	_____

Element	Meaning	Element	Meaning
51. cost-	_____	76. lobo-	_____
52. -gram	_____	77. -emesis	_____
53. acro-	_____	78. contra-	_____
54. rhexis	_____	79. -iasis	_____
55. carcin-	_____	80. trans-	_____
56. -penia	_____	81. brady-	_____
57. gen-	_____	82. -ectasis	_____
58. burso-	_____	83. cyt-	_____
59. retr(o)-	_____	84. odont-	_____
60. trip-	_____	85. leuk-	_____
61. strept-	_____	86. -esthesia	_____
62. -desis	_____	87. cantho-	_____
63. mani-	_____	88. steno-	_____
64. glosso-	_____	89. cheil-	_____
65. -trophy	_____	90. -cele	_____
66. supra-	_____	91. benign	_____
67. -ptosis	_____	92. semen	_____
68. -dyn-	_____	93. celio-	_____
69. mast-	_____	94. erythro-	_____
70. -rrhaphy	_____	95. vaso-	_____
71. dent-	_____	96. melan-	_____
72. cephal-	_____	97. cauda-	_____
73. auto-	_____	98. lingua-	_____
74. epi-	_____	99. myring-	_____
75. hydro-	_____	100. spondyl-	_____

Name _____

Element	Meaning	Element	Meaning
101. ovar-	_____	126. physio-	_____
102. -centesis	_____	127. bucc(o)-	_____
103. oto-	_____	128. palpebr-	_____
104. bili-	_____	129. -plasia	_____
105. squam-	_____	130. rug-	_____
106. mening-	_____	131. aur-	_____
107. cec-	_____	132. acoust(i)-	_____
108. macul-	_____	133. colp(o)-	_____
109. -pexy	_____	134. phon-	_____
110. onco-	_____	135. leio-	_____
111. or-	_____	136. cor	_____
112. sub-	_____	137. ren-	_____
113. spiro-	_____	138. orchi-	_____
114. lacrim-	_____	139. encephal-	_____
115. viscero-	_____	140. thalam-	_____
116. lact-	_____	141. plexus	_____
117. onych-	_____	142. cilia	_____
118. thorac-	_____	143. dendr-	_____
119. pyle-	_____	144. phleb-	_____
120. vesic-	_____	145. pilo-	_____
121. sphenic-	_____	146. histo-	_____
122. myel-	_____	147. stoma-	_____
123. anti-	_____	148. tympan-	_____
124. myco-	_____	149. umbilic-	_____
125. hallux	_____	150. salpingo-	_____

Element	Meaning	Element	Meaning
151. helio-	_____	176. pneum-	_____
152. astr-	_____	177. phage	_____
153. -asthenia	_____	178. phren-	_____
154. fascia	_____	179. corne-	_____
155. iso-	_____	180. plak-	_____
156. tarso-	_____	181. iris	_____
157. -tope	_____	182. kerat-	_____
158. pod-	_____	183. pulmon-	_____
159. malign-	_____	184. ptyal-	_____
160. adnexa	_____	185. alveol-	_____
161. ocul-	_____	186. oophor-	_____
162. lapar-	_____	187. oment-	_____
163. dacry-	_____	188. sedat-	_____
164. ment-	_____	189. furca-	_____
165. part-	_____	190. radic-	_____
166. scler(a)-	_____	191. radi-	_____
167. somato-	_____	192. fistul-	_____
168. trachel-	_____	193. edema	_____
169. sinus	_____	194. dactyl-	_____
170. hypno-	_____	195. metabol(e)-	_____
171. sept-	_____	196. pariet-	_____
172. scirr(h)-	_____	197. ependym-	_____
173. antr-	_____	198. gravid	_____
174. -crine	_____	199. aer-	_____
175. dura	_____	200. glyco-	_____

Name _____

Element	Meaning	Element	Meaning
201. tarso-	_____	226. mechano-	_____
202. cheir-, chir-	_____	227. dynam-	_____
203. calc-	_____	228. osmo-	_____
204. cine-	_____	229. traumat-	_____
205. digit	_____	230. trich-	_____
206. dors-	_____	231. maxill-	_____
207. gangli-	_____	232. an-, a-	_____
208. gemin-	_____	233. phak-	_____
209. grad-	_____	234. pre-	_____
210. gran-	_____	235. strict-	_____
211. labi-	_____	236. turbin-	_____
212. micr-	_____	237. ameb-	_____
213. peps-	_____	238. semi-	_____
214. pleur-	_____	239. neo-	_____
215. mamm-	_____	240. hormone	_____
216. colla-	_____	241. therm-	_____
217. later-	_____	242. syn-, sym-	_____
218. rachi-	_____	243. vuls-	_____
219. phob-	_____	244. post	_____
220. phot-	_____	245. metr-	_____
221. dys-	_____	246. tegument	_____
222. cut-	_____	247. pan-	_____
223. en-	_____	248. poly-	_____
224. peri-	_____	249. ramus	_____
225. pro-	_____	250. neuro-	_____

Element	Meaning	Element	Meaning
251. thromb-		276. arter-	
252. ab-		277. appendic-	
253. -plegia		278. thyro-	
254. ante-		279. splen-	
255. thel-		280. ovario-	
256. ex-		281. adreno-	
257. lien-		282. basi-	
258. tumor		283. pelvi-	
259. vestibule		284. vena-	
260. puer-		285. urethr-	
261. sarc-		286. utero-	
262. proli-		287. sacro-	
263. macro-		288. pharyng-	
264. lal-		289. duodeno-	
265. intra-		290. ureter-	
266. inter-		291. laryng-	
267. infra-		292. bronch-	
268. cryo-		293. col-	
269. mal-		294. esophag-	
270. glom-		295. bi-	
271. tens-		296. tri-	
272. spas-		297. ile-	
273. somni-		298. ili-	
274. pharmac-		299. lig-	
275. lumbo-		300. therap-	

Name _____

Element	Meaning	Element	Meaning
301. ventr-	_____	326. proxim-	_____
302. vert-	_____	327. scol-	_____
303. eu-	_____	328. apo-	_____
304. ambi-	_____	329. di-	_____
305. amphi-	_____	330. dia-	_____
306. brachy-	_____	331. eury-	_____
307. capit-	_____	332. pect-	_____
308. cau-	_____	333. necr-	_____
309. clas-	_____	334. mi-	_____
310. duct-	_____	335. morph-	_____
311. fiss-	_____	336. dis-	_____
312. ger-	_____	337. fac-	_____
313. heter-	_____	338. lept-	_____
314. infer-	_____	339. lymph-	_____
315. hom-	_____	340. meta-	_____
316. olfact-	_____	341. -rrhag	_____
317. orth-	_____	342. sta-	_____
318. gyn-	_____	343. ton-	_____
319. pachy-	_____	344. volv-	_____
320. phrag-	_____	345. splanchn-	_____
321. poster-	_____	346. -rrhe	_____
322. cata-	_____	347. med-	_____
323. platy-	_____	348. xer-	_____
324. pseud-	_____	349. per-	_____
325. schiz-	_____	350. blast-	_____

Introduction

THE DEAN VAUGHN TOTAL RETENTION SYSTEM™

This unique instructional system was developed by Dean Vaughn, who is recognized as the foremost authority in applied memory technology for learning. His instructional systems are used throughout the world in thousands of the finest academic, health, and business institutions with unprecedented success. This proven system of mnemonic instruction and learning has been acclaimed by educators as one of the most significant breakthroughs in education today.

As a student of medical terminology, you are fortunate to have the opportunity to use this organized system of applied memory techniques to learn the subject. It will teach you not only how to learn but also how to remember what you learn!

Countless others have had to learn medical terminology through the conventional method of repetition which is time consuming, tedious, and inefficient. It discourages rather than encourages the learning process. As an active participant in this unique and enjoyable learning experience, you will learn quickly and remember what you learn with ease and self-confidence.

The Dean Vaughn Total Retention System™ (The System) is designed to dramatically increase your ability to mentally store, process, and retrieve information. It works in conjunction with the natural learning process of your brain to remember infinitely more of what you see than what you hear or read. Your brain processes images of familiar and real objects faster and much easier than it does abstract information, information that is hard to conceive or understand. The majority of elements you must learn to master medical terminology are abstract or unfamiliar. As such, they are extremely difficult to learn. The Dean Vaughn Total Retention System™ converts the abstract information for you into images of real and familiar objects and associates them with the subject in such a way that makes it incredibly easy to learn and remember.

The success of this advanced instructional system is the result of over thirty years of continued research, development, testing, and classroom validation.

DESIRE

The most important ingredient to assure your success in this course is your desire to learn medical terminology. Without it, this course will be no more effective than any other. But with the desire, this course will not only be more effective but it will also be the most phenomenal and rewarding academic achievement you may ever experience. You will very quickly and easily learn what so many others have been unable to learn after hundreds of hours of difficult and frustrating study. Now, prepare yourself for a learning adventure. Be positive, work with The System, and The System will work for you!

PURPOSE OF THIS COURSE

The purpose of this course is to teach you the basic design of medical terminology and *how to easily remember* the meanings of 350 Latin and Greek word parts or elements. After successfully completing this course, you will be able to easily interpret and understand more than eleven thousand complex medical terms. This skill and ability will provide you with a powerful foundation of knowledge for the language of medicine.

IMPORTANCE OF THE LESSON PRESENTATION

Each of the fourteen lessons in this course is presented in a video format. Incorporated into each is the application of the Dean Vaughn Total Retention System™, a proven system of effective memory techniques, to teach you *how to easily remember* the simplified meanings of the 350 elements. The audio narration will guide you through the learning process in each lesson and will provide you with the pronunciations of the elements and the opportunity to practice them.

You will be asked not to take any notes during the presentation. It is essential that you concentrate totally on the lesson presentation and the application of the learning system. Because part of the system's memory technique is based on sound-a-like terminology, it is important that you pronounce the terms along with the narrator as directed. Your success in this course will depend primarily on your ability to remember and recall the sound-a-like terms.

> As you participate with the presentation, please understand that the cartoon images and their associations are used to depict illogical, unreal, and in many instances, ridiculous situations. This is done solely for their strong impressionistic values to aid you in mentally retaining and recalling the information. *They are not intended in any way to be insulting, insensitive, or indicative of any real life situation, person, place, or thing.*

IMPORTANCE OF THIS LEARNING GUIDE

This Learning Guide interacts closely with each video lesson presentation. It provides the following functions and exercises required to successfully complete the Dean Vaughn Total Retention System™ applied to Medical Terminology:

LESSON REVIEW - reviews the twenty-five medical elements taught in each lesson, their sound-a-like words (audionyms), illogical associations, and simplified meanings.

WORK SHEET EXERCISE - enables you to test yourself on the application of the learning system and the meanings of the twenty-five elements taught in each lesson.

WORD TERMINALS - teaches the meanings of many word endings used in medical terms by relating them to familiar English words.

READING ASSIGNMENT - expands the meanings of the twenty-five elements taught in each lesson. It shows the various forms in which they may be used in medical terms. The reading assignment explains the relationship of the elements with each other and when relevant, their functions, structures, and anatomical locations. Included are examples of each element's use in medical terms.

ELEMENT RECOGNITION EXERCISE - tests your skill in identifying lesson elements within complex medical terms.

INTERPRETATION EXERCISE - enables you to test yourself in interpreting medical terms comprised of lesson elements.

After completing the course, this Learning Guide will be a valuable reference for you. Use it routinely to review the system's application and confirm your retention of the 350 elements and their meanings.

PREVIOUS EDITION SUBSTITUTION PAGES

These five labeled sheets are located in this book immediately following the sheets containing Lesson Review Pages 50, 51, 88, 139, and 215, and are to be substituted when using this book with any pre-second edition audio-visual lesson. (That is any audio-visual program lesson having a copyright date before 2004.)

THE 100% AWARD FOR EXCELLENCE

This award is presented to those who satisfactorily complete this course and achieve a perfect score of one hundred percent on the final test.* Because this course has been designed for total retention of all the elements taught, it should be your objective to achieve this goal. The award will give evidence of your complete knowledge and understanding of medical terminology as presented in this course and will be a testament of your high academic achievement.

HOW TO ACHIEVE 100% ON YOUR FINAL TEST

1. Pay close attention and carefully participate with the audiovisual presentation of each lesson as directed.
2. During the presentation, be sure to pronounce each element, its sound-a-like word (audionym, as it is called by The System), and its meaning along with the narrator. It is important to pronounce the words aloud. If this is not possible, pronounce them in an almost silent whisper.
3. After each lesson presentation, complete the Lesson Review Exercise provided in this Learning Guide. Carefully review each element and picture in your mind its associated image as depicted in the video lesson's presentation.
4. After reviewing the lesson, complete its Work Sheet Exercise provided on the following page. Be sure to perform each step of the learning system in recalling the meaning of the element.
5. If you have difficulty in the Work Sheet Exercise recalling the meaning of an element or its associated learning steps, go back and review that element again.
6. After completing all fourteen lesson presentations and their corresponding Learning Guide activities, perform a final review of all 350 elements.
7. Always use these steps to recall a meaning: *Pronounce* the element; *Think* of the audionym; *Picture* the illogical association; *Recall* the meaning.

   (Suggestion: have a friend or fellow student quiz you in your knowledge of the 350 elements before taking the final test)

The use of the Dean Vaughn Learning System will enable you to quickly remember and effectively apply the 350 elements taught in this course. Eventually, as you become more familiar with them, it will be unnecessary for you to use The System. Do not try to rush the process. Always use The System to recall and confirm the meaning of a word or element within a medical term until the meaning is permanently established in your mind.

* Presented solely at the discretion of the provider of this course to you.

Important Definitions

MEDICAL TERM   a word or phrase made up of a combination of elements to express a specific idea

Example:

Element	+	Element	+	Element	Medical Term
hemi	+	*gastr*	+	*ectomy*	hemigastrectomy

ELEMENT   a word part used to form a medical term. All elements in a medical term are essential to its meaning. Each element in a medical term has its own meaning.

PREFIX   an element used at the beginning of a medical term which changes in some manner the meaning of the medical term or makes it more specific.

ROOT   the main element within a medical term. Often there is more than one root element within the medical term. The root element is always the subject or main topic of the medical term and is frequently a body part.

SUFFIX   an element used at the end of a medical term (after the root element) that frequently describes a condition of a body part or an action to a body part.

Example				
	Prefix	Root	Suffix	Medical Term
Element:	*hemi-* +	*gastr-* +	*-ectomy* =	hemigastrectomy
Meaning:	half	stomach	surgical removal	surgical removal of half the stomach

WORD
TERMINAL
a suffix or word ending that denotes the part of speech of the medical term (noun, verb, adjective).

The following word terminals are used in your everyday vocabulary. They will be used in your reading assignments:

Adjective terminals (pertaining to)	Noun terminals
-ic	-y
-al	-ia
-ical	-um
-ac	-is
	-a (ae—plural)

COMBINING
VOWEL
(usually **o** or **i** and, less frequently **u**) used between two elements of a medical term to make the term easier to pronounce. Occasionally the other vowels may be used

Example:

without combining vowel: gastrenteric (gastr/enter/ic)
with combining vowel: gastroenteric (gastr/o/enter/ic)

COMBINING
FORM
a root with an added combining vowel which the root usually carries when used in combination with another element

Example:

Root	+	Combining Vowel	=	Combining Form	+	Another Element	=	Medical Term
gastr		o		gastro		*enteric*		gastroenteric
(means)		*(for ease of pronunciation)*		(means)		(means)		(means)
stomach				stomach		pertaining to the intestines		pertaining to the intestines and stomach

☞ **Note:** You will notice that we teach certain basic root elements in their combining forms. We do so because of their frequent use and familiarity in medical terminology.

Lesson 1

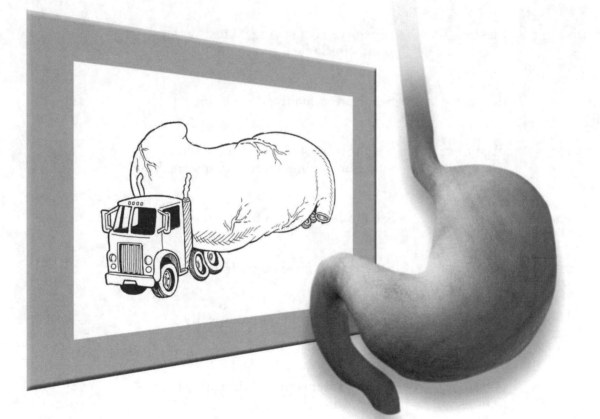

Element	Audionym	Visual Image	Meaning
gastr-	gas truck	See the **gas truck** with a **stomach** for a tank!	stomach
cardi-	card	See the people playing **card**s with real live **heart**s!	heart
megal-	my gal	See **my gal** as the most **enlarged** gal in the world!	enlarged
-itis	I test	See the teacher saying, "**I tes**t" as she stands **in flame**s!	inflammation
dermat-	doormat	See the **doormat** made of **skin**!	skin
plast-	plastic (plastic cement)	See the tube of **plast**ic cement with a **surgeon** coming out to **repair** something!	surgical repair
cerebr-	zebra	See the **zebra** with a **brain** for a head!	brain
path-	path	See the **path** covered with **daisies**!	disease
-ectomy	exit Tommy	See the **exit Tom**my is **surgically removing**!	surgical removal
enter-	enter (enter sign)	See the **enter** sign with **intestines** all over it!	intestines (usually small)
-osis	Oh Sis	See "**Oh Sis!**" holding the **air-conditio**ner!	any condition
-otomy	Oh Tommy	See Tommy's mother saying, "**Oh Tom**my! you **cut into** the wall!"	cut into

Lesson 1—Review

Element	Audionym	Visual Image	Meaning
aden-	a den	See **a den** with **gland**s hanging on the walls!	gland
angi-	angel	See the **ange**l covered with blood **vessel**s!	vessel
-oma	Oh Ma	See the children saying, **"Oh Ma!, two more!"**	tumor
nephr-	nephew	See the **neph**ew, a **kid** on the k**nee**!	kidney
hepat-	he pat	See the man as **he pat**s the **liver**!	liver
arthr-	art	See the **art** with **joint**s all over it!	joint
blephar-	blue fur	See the lady wearing a **blue fur** covered with **eyelid**s!	eyelid
-ologist	hollow chest	See the man with the h**ollow chest** for books: He is a **specialist**!	specialist
rhin-	rhinoceros	See the **rhin**oceros with a human **nose** growing on it!	nose
gingiv-	gingerbread (gingerbread man)	See the **ginger**bread man with **gum** stuck to him!	gum
-malacia	my late show (TV)	See the image for **my la**te **sh**ow, a TV that is very **soft**!	soft
-ology	hollow cheese	See the h**ollow che**ese with the people making a **study of** it!	the study of
spasm	spaceman	See the **space**man being forced to sign an **involuntary contract**!	involuntary contraction

Lesson 1—Worksheet

Print the audionym and meaning of the elements in the proper blanks:

Element	Audionym	Meaning
gastr-	gas truck	stomach
cardi-	cards	heart
megal-	my gal	enlarged
-itis	i test - in flames	inflamation
dermat-	doormat	skin
plast-	plastic cement	surgical repair
cerebr-	zebra	brain
path-	path - daisies	disease
-ectomy	exit tomy	surgically remove
enter-	enter sign	intestines
-osis	oh sis	any condition
-otomy	oh tomy	cut into
aden-	a den	gland
angi-	angle	vessel
-oma	oh ma	tumor
nephr-	nephew	kidney
hepat-	he pat	liver
arthr-	art	joint
blephar-	blue fur	eyelid
-ologist	hollow chest	specialist
rhin-	rhino	nose
gingiv-	gingerbread man	gum
-malacia	my late show	soft
-ology	hollow cheese	the study of
spasm	space man	involentary contractions

-ic, -al, -ac ✳	pertaining to

These terminals mean "pertaining to" when attached to a root or a combination of elements. Included under the meaning "pertaining to" are such ideas as:

"of or belonging to or having to do with" (histor/ic)
"of the nature of" (angel/ic, hero/ic)
"connected with" (athlet/ic, artist/ic)

☞ **Note:** The terminal -ac is not as widely used, either in common English or medical words, as are the -ic, -al, -ical terminals
Example: cardiac (cardi/ac)—"connected with the heart"; "of the heart"

-ical ✳	combination of -ic and -al but carries the same meaning "pertaining to" as set forth above under -ic, -al and -ac.

Example:
• mathemat/ical, method/ical, pract/ical, geograph/ical

-y ✳	the act of or result of an action; a condition or quality

Examples:
• dreamy (dream/y)—the condition or quality of exhibiting a dreamlike state
• inquiry (inquir/y)—the act of or result of asking questions (inquiring)

-ia ✳	a disease; an unhealthy state or condition

This terminal is widely used to name diseases such as dipther/ia, pneumon/ia, leukem/ia.

It may also be used to denote an unhealthy (morbid) condition such as:
• amnesia (amnes/ia)—loss of memory
• anesthesia (anesthes/ia)—loss of feeling
• phobia (phob/ia)—abnormal fear

-um ✳	noun ending; used to form the name of a thing from the root

Examples:
• addendum (addend/um)—something added
• momentum (moment/um)—something moving; a force

-is ✳ noun ending; used to form the name of a thing from the root

Example:
- dermis (derm/is)—the skin

Overcoming Problems
of Literal Interpretations

Since the majority of medical terms used in the practice of medicine are compound English derivatives of Latin and Greek words or parts of words, it is impossible to always have word for word or part of word translation or similarity in their interpretation.

To be certain that you are accurately interpreting a medical term, it will be necessary at times to refer to an authoritative medical dictionary. Failure to do this may result in an inaccurate interpretation.

Example:
cardiectomy (cardi = heart, ectomy = surgical removal of all or part of); therefore one might reasonably (but inaccurately) assume that cardiectomy means surgical removal of all or part of the heart. To quote one authoritative source, cardiectomy means "surgical removal of the upper end of the stomach or the portion closest to the heart..." Cardiectomized, however, means having the heart surgically removed.

☞   **Note:**   "Cardia" is the name given to the opening of the esophagus into the stomach. The meaning of this medical term was probably derived from the fact that the upper end of the stomach is the cardiac end or the end toward the end of the heart. In any case, it clearly emphasizes the importance of referring to an authoritative medical dictionary when needed rather than accepting the literal interpretation of a medical term.

aden- a gland; a body part that separates certain elements and secretes them in a form for the body to use or for elimination (e.g. sweat, urine)

Examples of glands:

Gland	Secretion
kidney	urine
mammary (mamm = breast)	milk
salivary	saliva

Examples:

- adenic (aden/ic)—pertaining to a gland or the glands
- adenopathy (aden/o/path/y)—any disease of a gland
- adenectomy (aden/ectomy)—surgical removal (excision) of all or part of a gland
- adenosis (aden/osis)—any condition of a gland
- adenotomy (aden/otomy)—cutting into (incision of) a gland
- adenoma (aden/oma)—a tumor with a glandlike structure (a glandular tumor)

☞ *Important: *Adenoma* does *not* mean tumor of a gland. An *adenoma* is a tumor with a glandlike structure (a glandular tumor) of any body part.

Examples of adenoma:

- blepharadenoma (blephar/aden/oma)—a glandular tumor of the eyelid (an adenoma of the eyelid)
- nephradenoma (nephr/aden/oma)—a glandular tumor of the kidney (an adenoma of the kidney)

angi- This element means "vessel" and therefore may be used to designate any of the tubes, ducts or canals that convey the fluids of the body. However, its principal reference is to a blood vessel or the blood vessels.

Examples:

- angiitis (angi/itis)—inflammation of a vessel or vessels—usually a blood vessel
- angiectomy (angi/ectomy)—surgical removal of a vessel or vessels
- angiomegaly (angi/o/megal/y)—enlargement of a vessel or vessels
- angiopathy (angi/o/path/y)—any disease of a vessel or vessels
- angiomalacia (angi/o/malacia)—softening of a vessel or vessels
- angiosis (angi/osis)—any condition of a vessel or vessels

☞ **Note**: The suffix element *-osis* is often used to denote a disease; therefore, angiosis could also mean any disease of the vessels.

arthr-   a joint; a joint of the body; the point where two bones come together

Examples:

- arthral (arthr/al)—pertaining to a joint
- arthritis (arthr/itis)—inflammation of a joint
- arthrotomy (arthr/otomy)—cutting into or incision of a joint
- arthrosis (arthr/osis)—any condition or disease of a joint
- arthropathy (arthr/o/path/y)—any disease of a joint

blephar-   the eyelid

Examples:

- blepharal (blephar/al)—pertaining to the eyelid
- blepharoplasty (blephar/o/plast/y)—plastic repair or surgery of an eyelid
- blepharospasm (blephar/o/spasm)— involuntary contractions of the eyelid
- blepharadenoma (blephar/aden/oma)—a glandular tumor of the eyelid
- blepharitis (blephar/itis)—inflammation of an eyelid
- blepharectomy (blephar/ectomy)—surgical removal (excision) of all or part of the eyelid

cardi-   the heart

Examples:

- cardiac (cardi/ac)—pertaining to the heart
- cardiopathy (cardi/o/path/y)—any disease of the heart
- carditis (card/itis)— inflammation of the heart
- cardiology (cardi/ology)— the study of the heart
- cardiologist (cardi/ologist)—a specialist in the study of the heart
- cardiomegaly (cardi/o/megal/y)—enlargement of the heart
- cardiomalacia (cardi/o/malacia)—softening of the heart
- cardiotomy (cardi/otomy)—cutting into (incision) of the heart

cerebr-   the brain

Examples:

- cerebral (cerebr/al)—pertaining to the brain
- cerebrum (cerebr/um)—the main part of the brain
- cerebritis (cerebr/itis)—inflammation of the brain
- cerebrospinal (cerebr/o/spin/al)—pertaining to the brain and the spinal cord
- cerebrosis (cerebr/osis)—any condition or disease of the brain
- cerebromalacia (cerebr/o/malacia)—softening of the brain
- cerebrology (cerebr/ology)—the study of the brain
- cerebropathy (cerebr/o/path/y)—any disease of the brain

dermat-   (also derm-) the skin

Examples:
- dermal (derm/al)—pertaining to the skin
- dermatic (dermat/ic)—pertaining to the skin
- dermic (derm/ic)—pertaining to the skin
- derma (derm/a)—the skin
- dermis (derm/is)—the skin
- dermatitis (dermat/itis)—inflammation of the skin
- dermatomegaly (dermat/o/megal/y)— enlargement of the skin; a condition in which the skin is larger than is necessary to cover the body so that it hangs in folds
- dermatosis (dermat/osis)—any condition or disease of the skin
- dermatopathy (dermat/o/path/y)—any disease of the skin
- dermatoplasty (dermat/o/plast/y)— plastic repair or surgery on the skin such as skin grafting
- dermatology (dermat/ology)—the study of the skin
- dermatologist (dermat/ologist)—a specialist in the study of the skin
- dermabrasion (derm/abrasion)—a scraping of the skin in order to repair acne scars, blemishes, etc.

-ectomy   Surgical removal (excision) of all or part of a body part. This suffix is used frequently in medical terminology and can be applied to almost any body part.

Examples:
- adenectomy (aden/ectomy)—surgical removal of a gland
- angiectomy (angi/ectomy)—surgical removal of a vessel
- arthrectomy (arthr/ectomy)—surgical removal of a joint
- blepharectomy (blephar/ectomy)—surgical removal of an eyelid
- enterectomy (enter/ectomy)—surgical removal of the intestines
- gastrectomy (gastr/ectomy)—surgical removal of the stomach
- nephrectomy (nephr/ectomy)—surgical removal of the kidney

enter-   the intestines; the approximate 6 meter (20 foot) long tube in the abdomen that completes the digestion of food begun in the stomach

Examples:
- enteral (enter/al)—pertaining to the intestines
- enteric (enter/ic)—pertaining to the intestines
- gastroenter- (gastr/o/enter-)—the stomach and intestines
- enteritis (enter/itis)—inflammation of the intestines
- enterectomy (enter/ectomy)—excision of a part of the intestines
- enteropathy (enter/o/path/y)—any disease of the intestines
- enteroplasty (enter/o/plast/y)—plastic repair or surgery of the intestines
- enteraden- (enter/aden-)—any gland of the intestines
- enteradenitis (enter/aden/itis)—inflammation of the glands of the intestines

gastr- the stomach; the balloon-like organ in the abdomen that begins the digestion of food

Examples:
- gastric (gastr/ic)—pertaining to the stomach
- gastrointestinal (gastr/o/intestin/al) system—the digestive system; the combination of the stomach and intestines responsible for the digestion of food
- gastroenteric (gastr/o/enter/ic)—pertaining to the stomach and intestines; pertaining to the digestive system
- gastradenitis (gastr/aden/itis)—inflammation of the glands of the stomach
- gastrectomy (gastr/ectomy)—surgical removal of the whole or part of the stomach
- partial gastrectomy—excision of a large portion but not all of the stomach

gingiv- gum; the gums of the mouth; the tissue that forms the collar around each tooth

Examples:
- gingival (gingiv/al)—pertaining to the gums
- gingiva (gingiv/a)—gum of the mouth
- gingivae (gingiv/ae)—gums of the mouth
- gingivitis (gingiv/itis)—inflammation of the gums of the mouth
- gingivectomy (gingiv/ectomy)—excision of the gums of the mouth
- gingivoplasty (gingiv/o/plast/y)—plastic repair or surgery of the gums of the mouth

hepat- the liver; the largest gland in the body, weighing about 1.5 kilograms (3 pounds); secretes bile into the intestine for digestion of fats

Examples:
- hepatic (hepat/ic)—pertaining to the liver
- hepatitis (hepat/itis)—inflammation of the liver
- hepatology (hepat/ology)—the study of the liver
- hepatologist (hepat/ologist)—a specialist in the study of the liver
- hepatomegaly (hepat/o/megal/y)—enlargement of the liver
- hepatonephritis (hepat/o/nephr/itis)—inflammation of the liver and kidney
- hepatonephromegaly (hepat/o/nephr/o/megal/y)—enlargement of the liver and kidney
- hepatectomy (hepat/ectomy)—excision of part of the liver
- hepatomalacia (hepat/o/malacia)—softening of the liver

-itis inflammation; "inflammation of—"; a suffix indicating a condition, the symptoms of which are pain or discomfort, redness, heat, and swelling. This suffix can be added to practically all body parts. Notice how rapidly your knowledge of medical terminology expands simply by adding this suffix to the elements of Lesson 1.

Examples:

- gastritis (gastr/itis)—inflammation of the stomach
- carditis (card/itis)— inflammation of the heart
- dermatitis (dermat/itis)—inflammation of the skin
- cerebritis (cerebr/itis)—inflammation of the brain (cerebrum)
- enteritis (enter/itis)—inflammation of the intestines
- adenitis (aden/itis)—inflammation of a gland or glands
- angiitis (angi/itis)—inflammation of the vessels
- angitis (ang/itis)—inflammation of the vessels
- nephritis (nephr/itis)—inflammation of the kidney
- hepatitis (hepat/itis)—inflammation of the liver
- arthritis (arthr/itis)—inflammation of a joint
- blepharitis (blephar/itis)—inflammation of the eyelid
- rhinitis (rhin/itis)—inflammation of the nose
- gingivitis (gingiv/itis)— inflammation of the gums of the mouth
- angiocarditis (angi/o/card/itis)—inflammation of the heart and blood vessels
- blepharadenitis (blephar/aden/itis)—inflammation of the glands of the eyelid
- enteradenitis (enter/aden/itis)—inflammation of the glands of the intestines
- enterogastritis (enter/o/gastr/itis)—inflammation of the intestine (small) and the stomach
- enterohepatitis (enter/o/hepat/itis)—inflammation of the intestines and the liver
- gastradenitis (gastr/aden/itis)—inflammation of the glands of the stomach
- gastrohepatitis (gastr/o/hepat/itis)—inflammation of the stomach and liver
- gastroenteritis (gastr/o/enter/itis)—inflammation of the stomach and intestines
- gastronephritis (gastr/o/nephr/itis)—inflammation of the stomach and kidney
- hepatonephritis (hepat/o/nephr/itis)—inflammation of the liver and kidney

-malacia   soft, soft condition, softness, softening. All body parts have a characteristically normal firmness; abnormal lessening of this firmness is denoted by malacia.

A suffix denoting a condition of softness; this is the form in which the term most frequently appears as in:

- adenomalacia (aden/o/malacia)—softening of a gland
- cardiomalacia (cardi/o/malacia)— softening of the heart
- cerebromalacia (cerebr/o/malacia)—softening of the brain (cerebrum)
- hepatomalacia (hepat/o/malacia)—softening of the liver
- nephromalacia (nephr/o/malacia)—softening of the kidney

In structures that are hollow such as vessels or the stomach, softening would be present in the walls of the structure, for example:

- angiomalacia (angi/o/malacia)—softening of the walls of a blood vessel
- gastromalacia (gastr/o/malacia)—softening of the walls of the stomach

megal- enlarged, literally "pertaining to largeness," "enlargement of—," but used principally to denote abnormal size. Body parts have a characteristically normal size related to age, sex, body type, etc. Abnormal increases in size are denoted by "*megal-*."

Examples:

-megaly (megal/y) is the form in which "enlarged" most frequently appears, for example:

- adenomegaly (aden/o/megal/y)—enlargement of a gland
- angiomegaly (angi/o/megal/y)—enlargement of a blood vessel
- cardiomegaly (cardi/o/megal/y)—enlargement of the heart
- cerebromegaly (cerebr/o/megal/y)—enlargement of the brain (cerebrum)
- enteromegaly (enter/o/megal/y)—enlargement of the intestines
- gastromegaly (gastr/o/megal/y)—enlargement of the stomach
- hepatomegaly (hepat/o/megal/y)—enlargement of the liver
- nephromegaly (nephr/o/megal/y)—enlargement of a kidney
- cardiohepatomegaly (cardi/o/hepat/o/megal/y)—enlargement of the heart and liver

megalo- (megal/o) is another form for "enlarged." The format indicating abnormal condition of enlargement is "megalo_____ia." For example:

- megalocardia (megal/o/card/ia)—abnormal enlargement of the heart
- megalogastria (megal/o/gastr/ia)—abnormal enlargement of the stomach
- megalohepatia (megal/o/hepat/ia)—abnormal enlargement of the liver

nephr- a kidney, the kidneys; the kidneys consist of two bean-shaped glands in the lower back, one on each side of the spinal column. Their function is the filtering of waste materials from the blood and the production and excretion of urine.

Examples:

- nephric (nephr/ic)—pertaining to the kidneys
- nephromegaly (nephr/o/megal/y)—enlargement of a kidney
- nephritis (nephr/itis)—inflammation of a kidney
- nephrosis (nephr/osis)—any condition of a kidney
- nephroma (nephr/oma)—tumor of the kidney
- nephropathy (nephr/o/path/y)—any disease of a kidney
- nephrotomy (nephr/otomy)— surgical cutting into (incision) of a kidney
- nephrectomy (nephr/ectomy)—surgical cutting out (excision) of all or part of a kidney
- nephrology (nephr/ology)—study of the kidneys
- nephrologist (nephr/ologist)—a specialist in the study of the kidneys
- nephradenoma (nephr/aden/oma)—glandular tumor of a kidney
- hepatonephromegaly (hepat/o/nephr/o/megal/y)—enlargement of the liver and kidney

-ologist   a specialist in the study of—; a medical specialist in—; one who has knowledge of or skill in—; an expert—

Examples:
- gastrologist (gastr/ologist)—a specialist in the study of the stomach
- cardiologist (cardi/ologist)—a specialist in the study of the heart
- dermatologist (dermat/ologist)—a specialist in the study of the skin
- enterologist (enter/ologist)—a specialist in the study of the intestines
- nephrologist (nephr/ologist)—a specialist in the study of the kidneys
- hepatologist (hepat/ologist)— a specialist in the study of the liver
- rhinologist (rhin/ologist)—a specialist in the study of the nose
- gastroenterologist (gastr/o/enter/ologist)—a specialist in the study of the stomach and intestines
- pathologist (path/ologist)—a specialist in the study of diseases

-ology   study of; knowledge of; especially "the science of"; a specialized department of medicine; a specialized field of medical practice

This suffix is used widely in medicine to name the field in which a physician may decide to limit his practice, particularly if he has undergone training and examination in the field.

Examples:
- dermatology (dermat/ology)—the branch of medicine dealing with the skin and its disorders
- pathology (path/ology)—the branch of medicine that deals with the nature of disease

Internal medicine—the branch of medicine that deals with the diagnosis and nonsurgical treatment of disease. Within this branch are specialized fields termed subspecialties.

These include:
- cardiology (cardi/ology)—the field of medicine dealing with the heart, its functions and its diseases
- nephrology (nephr/ology)—the field of medicine dealing with the kidneys, their functions and their diseases
- gastroenterology (gastr/o/enter/ology)—the field of medicine concerned with disorders of the digestive system. This field may be further divided between the specialties of gastrology and enterology

-oma   a tumor; a swelling on some part of the body; especially a mass of new tissue growth

Most applications of this suffix have to do with the composition of the tumor, that is, the kind of tissue forming the tumor.

For example:
- cerebroma (cerebr/oma)—an abnormal mass of brain tissue
- dermatoma (dermat/oma)—an abnormal growth of skin tissue

The term may describe structural features, such as:
- adenoma (aden/oma)—a tumor with a glandlike structure
- angioma (angi/oma)—a tumor which tends to be made up of blood vessels
- blepharadenoma (blephar/aden/oma)—a tumor of the eyelid consisting of gland-like structures; a glandular tumor of the eyelid

The term may also indicate the location of the tumor, as in hepatoma (hepat/oma).

As you progress through subsequent lessons and learn the roots for other body materials such as blood, cancers, fat, etc., you will discover many more *-oma* words.

From this discussion we can conclude that the appearance of the suffix *-oma* can usually be interpreted as:
"a tumor composed of—"
"a tumor consisting of—"
"a tumor arising from—"

-osis   condition or disease; most frequently used to indicate an abnormal or diseased condition; sometimes used in words not relating to disease such as in hypnosis

Examples:
- gastrosis (gastr/osis)—a condition of the stomach
- dermatosis (dermat/osis)—a condition of the skin
- cerebrosis (cerebr/osis)—a condition of the brain (cerebrum)
- enterosis (enter/osis)—a condition of the intestines
- adenosis (aden/osis)—a condition of a gland
- angiosis (angi/osis)—a condition of a blood vessel
- nephrosis (nephr/osis)—a condition of a kidney
- hepatosis (hepat/osis)—a condition of the liver
- arthrosis (arthr/osis)—a condition of a joint
- acidosis (acid/osis)—a condition or disease of acid in the body

✳ **-otomy**   cutting into (surgical incision); literally "the act or action of cutting into"— usually for the purpose of exploration, drainage, removal of foreign bodies, etc.

Examples:
- adenotomy (aden/otomy)—surgical incision of a gland
- arthrotomy (arthr/otomy)—surgical incision of a joint
- enterotomy (enter/otomy)—surgical incision of the intestines
- gastrotomy (gastr/otomy)—surgical incision of the stomach
- hepatotomy (hepat/otomy)—surgical incision of the liver
- nephrotomy (nephr/otomy)—surgical incision of the kidney

✳ *path-*   disease; suffering; feeling

Examples:
- pathic (path/ic)—pertaining to disease or feeling
- pathology (path/ology)—the field of medicine specializing in the study of diseases
- pathosis (path/osis)—a condition of disease; *-pathy*

The *-pathy* suffix combines with many body parts to denote "any disease of—".

Examples:
- adenopathy (aden/o/path/y)—any disease of a gland
- angiopathy (angi/o/path/y)—any disease of a blood vessel
- arthropathy (arthr/o/path/y)—any disease of a joint
- cardiopathy (cardi/o/path/y)—any disease of the heart
- cerebropathy (cerebr/o/path/y)—any disease of the brain (cerebrum)
- dermopathy (derm/o/path/y)—any disease of the skin
- dermatopathy (dermat/o/path/y)—any disease of the skin
- enteropathy (enter/o/path/y)—any disease of the intestines
- gastropathy (gastr/o/path/y)—any disease of the stomach
- hepatopathy (hepat/o/path/y)—any disease of the liver
- nephropathy (nephr/o/path/y)—any disease of the kidneys
- rhinopathy (rhin/o/path/y)—any disease of the nose

The *-pathic* suffix combines with all of the roots listed under *-pathy* with the meaning "pertaining to any disease of—."

plast-   plastic repair; renewal of destroyed, injured or deformed tissue; reforming, reconstruction or restoration of destroyed, injured or deformed body parts

Some examples of plastic repair are:
- correction of congenital (birth) defects such as cleft lip, webbed fingers
- cosmetic (beautifying) operations such as face lifts, "nose alterations"

-plasty (plast/y)—"surgical repair of—"

Examples:
- angioplasty (angi/o/plast/y)—plastic repair of a blood vessel
- arthroplasty (arthr/o/plast/y)—plastic repair of a joint
- blepharoplasty (blephar/o/plast/y)—plastic repair of an eyelid
- cardioplasty (cardi/o/plast/y)—plastic repair of the heart
- dermoplasty (derm/o/plast/y)—plastic repair of the skin
- dermatoplasty (dermat/o/plast/y)—plastic repair of the skin
- enteroplasty (enter/o/plast/y)—plastic repair of the intestines
- gastroplasty (gastr/o/plast/y)—plastic repair of the stomach
- gingivoplasty (gingiv/o/plast/y)—plastic repair of the gums
- rhinoplasty (rhin/o/plast/y)—plastic repair of the nose

-plastic (plast/ic)—pertaining to surgical repair

The *-plastic* suffix combines with all the roots listed under *-plasty* with the meaning "pertaining to surgical repair."

rhin   the nose

Examples:
- rhinal (rhin/al)—pertaining to the nose (same as nasal)
- rhinoplasty (rhin/o/plast/y)—plastic repair of the nose; rebuilding, reconstruction of or forming the nose
- rhinitis (rhin/itis)—inflammation of the nose (inflammation of the mucous membrane of the nose)
- rhinology (rhin/ology)—the study of the nose
- rhinologist (rhin/ologist)—specialist in the study of the nose

-spasm   involuntary contraction(s); a sudden, violent, involuntary contraction of a muscle or group of muscles; a sudden but brief constriction of a body passage or opening; a convulsion is a series of severe spasms

Examples:
- Angiospasm (angi/o/spasm) and enterospasm (enter/o/spasm) are examples of body passage spasms.
- Blepharospasm (blephar/o/spasm) is an example of a muscle spasm since it is caused by contraction of the muscle governing movement of the eyelid.

Lesson 1—Element Recognition

Separate the word terminals, elements, and connecting vowels, of the following medical terms from right to left by inserting a slash mark (/) between them.

Example: hepatonephromegaly—hepat/o/nephr/o/megal/y

gastro/hepat/itis	hepatonephromegaly
adenopathy	blepharoplasty
cardiomegaly	rhinologist
enteroplasty	gingivectomy
dermatologist	arthritis
pathosis	enterogastritis
cerebromalacia	pathology
angiopathology	dermatoma
nephrologist	cardiomalacia
hepatitis	adenotomy
arthrectomy	arthroplasty
blepharospasm	angiology
rhinology	blepharotomy
gingivosis	gastritis
angiomegaly	pathologist
nephromalacia	adenectomy
hepatoma	gingivitis
cerebropathy	nephrotomy
gastrectomy	cerebritis
enteromegaly	rhinopathy
cardiology	dermatitis

Lesson 1—Interpretation Exercise

Complete the following statements by printing the meanings of the elements that make up the medical term in the proper blanks. Use the System to aid you. Pronounce the element, recall its audionym and picture its illogical association. Remember, most medical terms are interpreted from right to left.

Example:

Adenosis (aden/osis) is a term which refers to any _____ of a _____.

(interpreting from right to left)
osis sounds like oasis / see an oasis with air conditioners / osis means condition
aden sounds like a den / see a den with glands / aden means gland

Adenosis (aden/osis) is a term that refers to any _____*condition*_____ of a _____*gland*_____.

Keep in mind that the meanings of medical terms, as explained in the Reading Assignment, are not always literal interpretations of the combined meanings of their elements. However, they are in some way derived from, affiliated with, or are extensions of them.

1-1.   An adenectomy (aden/ectomy) is the surgical _____ of all or part of

a _____.

1-2.   The term angiopathy (angi/o/path/y) denotes any _____ of a _____.

1-3.   Arthritis (arthr/itis) is an _____ of a _____.

1-4.   Blepharoplasty (blephar/o/plast/y) denotes the surgical _____ of

an _____.

1-5.   A cardiologist (cardi/ologist) is a specialist in the _____ of the _____.

1-6.   The term cerebromalacia (cerebr/o/malacia) denotes a _____ of

the _____.

1-7.   Dermatitis (dermat/itis) is an _____ of the _____.

1-8.   A gastrectomy (gastr/ectomy) is the surgical _____ of all or part of

the _____.

1-9.   The term enteric (enter/ic) means pertaining to or of the _____.

1-10.   The term gastroenteric (gastr/o/enter/ic) pertains to the _____ and
        the _____.

1-11.   Gingivitis (gingiv/itis) is an _____ of the _____.

1-12.   Hepatology (hepat/ology) is the _____ of the _____.

1-13.   Gastroenteritis (gastr/o/enter/itis) is an _____ of the _____ and
        the _____.

1-14.   Nephromalacia (nephr/o/malacia) denotes a _____ of the _____.

1-15.   Hepatomegaly (hepat/o/megal/y) denotes an _____ of the _____.

1-16.   The term nephrosis (nephr/osis) refers to any _____ of the _____.

1-17.   A pathologist (path/ologist) is a specialist in the _____ of _____.

1-18.   Dermatology (dermat/ology) is the _____ of the _____ .

1-19.   An adenoma (aden/oma) is a _____ that has a _____ular structure.

1-20.   The term gastrosis (gastr/osis) indicates a _____ of the _____.

1-21.   A nephrotomy (nephr/otomy) is the surgical incision into
        the _____.

1-22.   The term cerebropathy (cerebr/o/path/y) refers to any _____ of
        the _____.

1-23.   Gingivoplasty (gingiv/o/plast/y) denotes the plastic or surgical _____ of
        the _____.

1-24.   Rhinal (rhin/al) is a term pertaining to or of the _____.

1-25.   An enterospasm (enter/o/spasm) is an involuntary _____ of the _____.

Lesson 2

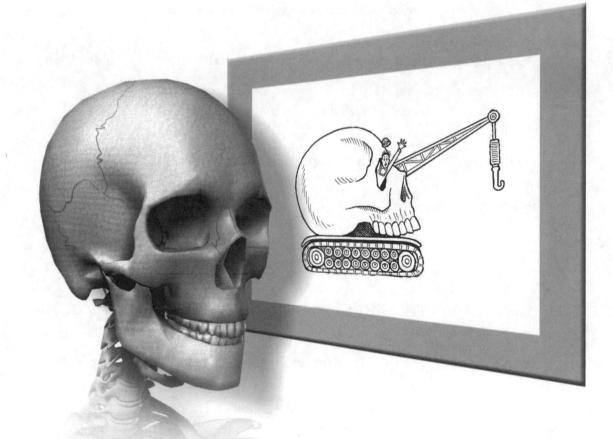

Lesson 2—Review

Element	Audionym	Visual Image	Meaning
-algia	algae	See the **algae** on the pond with a window **pane** floating on it!	pain
crani-	crane	See the **crane** made of a **skull**!	skull
end-	The End	See the **end** of the motion picture with real people **inside** or **within** the screen!	inside, within
hemi-	hemisphere	See the **hemi**sphere broken in **half**!	half
-oid	void	See the v**oid**ed checks that look a**like**!	like
hyper-	high purr	See the cat **high-purr**ing **above** a **more than normal** number of cats on the church!	above, more than normal
cyst-	sister	See **sist**er holding a **sack containing fluid**!	sac containing fluid
chole-	coal	See the **coal pile** on top of the coal!	bile
hypo-	hippo	See the **hippo under** the table!	under
-scop-	scope	See the tele**scop**e with people **observing** it, instead of looking through it!	observe
hyster-	his stir	See **his stir** saying, "Yo**u turn us**"!	uterus
-ostomy	Oh stop Tommy	See Tommy's mother saying, "**Oh sto**p Tom**my**!" as he runs away after **creating an opening** in the wall!	create an opening

Element	Audionym	Visual Image	Meaning
para-	parachute	See the **para**chutes **beside** each other and other **para**chutes **beyond** them!	beside, beyond
-lysis	license	See the **lic**ense **loosening** and being **destroyed**!	loosening, destruction
cervic-	serve hic	See the waiter **serv**ing **hic**cups from a bottle with a real **neck**!	neck
chondr-	cone door	See the **con**e with a **door** and a **cart of leaves** bursting out of it!	cartilage
cyan-	sign	See the stop **sign** with **blue** paint poured over it!	blue
hem(at)-	hem	See the **hem** with **blood** all over it!	blood
ost-	ostrich	See the **ost**rich made of **bone**s!	bone
psycho-	cycle	See the cycle with people fighting over it saying, **"Mine, Mine!"**	mind
lip-	lip	See the **lip** that is very **fat**!	fat
my-	my eye	See **my** eye with **muscles**!	muscle
lith-	lather	See the **lath**er on the man's face with a **stone** in it!	stone
ophthalm- opt-	up thumb	See the **up thum**b (thumbs up) with an **eye** on it!	eye
proct-	Procter & Gamble	See the **Proct**er & Gamble container with **Ana**cins pouring out of it!	anus

Lesson 2—Worksheet

Print the audionym and meaning of the elements in the proper blanks:

Element	Audionym	Meaning
-algia	alge	pain
crani-	crane	skull
end-	the end	inside, within
hemi-	hemisphere	half
-oid	void	like
hyper-	high purr	above, more then normal
cyst-	sister	sac containing fluid
chole-	coal	bile
hypo-	hippo	below
-scop-	scope	observe
hyster-	his stir	uterus
-ostomy	oh stop tommy	make an opening
para-	paracute	beside, beyond
-lysis	licence	loosening, destruction
cervic-	serve nick	neck
chondr-	cone dar	cartilage
cyan-	sign	blue
hem(at)-	hem	blood
ost-	ostrich	bone
psycho-	cycle	mind
lip-	lip	fat
my-	eye	muscle
lith-	lather	stone
ophthalm-	up thumb	eye
proct-		anus

Lesson 2—Word Terminals

-ar	pertaining to; having a connection with

Example:
- polar (pol/ar)—pertaining to the poles; a polar bear, a polar exploration

This "pertaining to" suffix is most frequently applied to words ending in *-l* or *-le* and is in the form *-ular*.

Examples:
- triangle—triang/ular; circle—circ/ular; muscle—musc/ular; single—sing/ular

-ary	pertaining to; having a connection with

Examples:
- honor/ary, budget/ary, unit/ary

✳ *-cle*	small; little

This terminal forms a "diminutive" that is the dictionary term for a word denoting a small version of the thing indicated by the main part of the word.

Examples:
- a part/i/cle is a "small part."
- an oss/i/cle is "a small bone."

✳ *-e*	means of; instrument for

This terminal is usually applied to action roots (verbs) to denote a means by which an action is performed, an instrument for performing the action.

Example:
- scope (scop/e)—a means of looking or observing; an instrument for looking or observing

A telescope (tele/scop/e) is an instrument for "looking or observing far away." (The element *tele-* means "distant, far away.") A telephone (tele/phon/e) is an instrument for "distant sound." (The element *phon-* means "sound" and is discussed in Lesson 6.)

-an, -ian	of or belonging to; frequently a person belonging to or associated with

Examples:
- Europe/an, Ohio/an, Florid/ian

| *-ide* | a terminal used in the naming of chemical compounds |

Examples:
- cyan/ide, brom/ide, chlor/ide

| ✳ *-ist* | one who practices; one who does; one who is concerned with |

Examples:
- organ/ist, machin/ist, humor/ist, novel/ist, chem/ist

| *-ium* | noun ending; frequently means place or region, lining or covering tissue |

See the reading assignment under the element *end-* for a specific discussion of the "tissue" meaning.

Examples:
- auditorium (auditor/ium)—a place for hearing
- podium (pod/ium)—a place for standing

| ✳ *-ule* | small, little; a diminutive (see *-cle* above) |

Examples:
- globule (glob/ule)—a tiny ball or globe
- capsule (caps/ule)—a small case or container
- venule (ven/ule)—a small vein

| *-ular* | (ul/ar) pertaining to (-ar) a small or little (-ul[e]); pertaining to a small version of the thing indicated by the main part of the word |

Example:
- valvular (valv/ular)—pertaining to a small valve

> ☞ **Note:** in separating and identifying word terminals you may experience some confusion in determining whether the *-ular* terminal is the combination of *-ul* (small) and *-ar* (pertaining to); or whether it has a "pertaining to" only meaning (see *-ar* above). The principal key is whether the main part of the word ends in *-l* or *-le* in which case the terminal has only the "pertaining to" meaning. The context (that is, the way in which the word is or can be used) will also serve to clarify the meaning. For example, it would not make sense to apply a diminutive (small, little) meaning to sing/ular; the idea of a "little single" is meaningless.

Lesson 2—Reading Assignment

-algia pain; painful condition; a sensation of hurting, or strong discomfort, in some part of the body caused by an injury, disease or malfunction of some body structure and transmitted through the nervous system

The suffix stem *-algia* can be attached to any part of the body containing nerves to denote the location of pain.

Examples:

- cerebralgia and cephalalgia (cerebr/algia, cephal/algia)—Note: Although *cerebr* means "brain" and *cephal* means "head," both cerebralgia and cephalalgia are used to denote "headache"—cephalalgia being the more common term
- arthralgia (arthr/algia)—pain in the joint(s)
- myalgia (my/algia)—pain in a muscle; muscle pain
- cardialgia (cardi/algia)—pain in the heart; heart pain
- gastralgia (gastr/algia)—pain in the stomach; stomach pain, stomach ache, "belly ache"

The element *-algia* may be further separated into two parts:

Literally (*-ia*) "condition of" (*alg-*) "pain,"— *-algia* is the most frequent form expressing pain. However, *alg-* is a root meaning "pain" and can appear in other forms such as *algesi-, algo-, algeo-,* and *algio-*.

Examples:

- algesi (alges/i)—form most frequently used to denote "sensitivity to pain"
- algesia (alges/ia)—sensitiveness to pain:
  - hyperalgesia (hyper/alges/ia)—excessive sensitiveness to pain
  - hypoalgesia (hypo/alges/ia)—abnormally low sensitivity to pain
- algesic (alges/ic)—pertaining to pain, painful
- algospasm (alg/o/spasm)—painful involuntary contraction; painful cramp
- algiomuscular (algi/o/muscular)—causing painful muscular movements; Note: remember myalgia (my/algia)—pain in the muscle

The use of the different forms for *alg-*, that is, *algo-, algeo-* and *algio-*, etc., is to avoid confusion with the form for *algae* which is the name for a group of plants, including seaweed and many fresh-water plants.

a or an - without

cervic- the neck or a neck-like structure

Examples:

- cervical (cervic/al)—pertaining to the cervix, neck or a neck-like structure
- cervicofacial (cervic/o/fac/i/al)—pertaining to the neck and face
- cervicoplasty (cervic/o/plast/y)—plastic surgery on the neck
- cervicitis (cervic/itis)—inflammation of the neck of the uterus (womb)

The cervical vertebrae are those bones of the spine that are located in the region of the neck.

The cervix (cerv/ix) is the name for the neck or a necklike part of the body; used to name those parts of the large bones of the body where the bone becomes narrow (constricted) behind the knoblike end (head). The narrow part of a tooth at the gumline is also called the cervix or "neck" of the tooth. The name is applied to the narrow (constricted) parts of pearshaped organs such as the uterus and the gall and urinary bladders.

chole-   bile; gall; yellow-brown or greenish fluid secreted by the liver and stored in the gallbladder (cholecyst)

The purpose of bile is to help in the digestion of foods, particularly fats. Bile is formed in and secreted from the liver (hepat-) and stored in the gallbladder (cholecyst) from where it is discharged through the bile duct (cholangi-) into the intestines (enter-).

Examples:
- choleic (chole/ic)—pertaining to or derived from the bile; "of the bile"; "from the bile"
- cholangi- (chol/angi-)—the bile vessel; the bile duct, the tube through which bile passes

☞   **Note:** Another name for the bile duct (sometimes called "the common bile duct" since it is a duct which is common to [joins] the liver and gallbladder) is *choledoch-*.

- cholecyst (chole/cyst)—the bile sac; the bile bladder; the gallbladder (gall and bile are synonyms); the storage "bag" for bile (gall) after it is manufactured in the liver and before it is needed by the intestine
- cholangitis (chol/ang/itis)—inflammation of a bile duct (bile vessel)
  From Lesson 1 Reading Assignment: ". . . this element actually means 'vessel' and, therefore, may be used to designate any of the tubes, ducts or canals which convey the fluids of the body."
- cholecystectomy (chole/cyst/ectomy)—surgical removal (excision) of the gallbladder
- cholecystalgia (chole/cyst/algia)—pain in the gallbladder
- cholecystitis (chole/cyst/itis)—inflammation of the gallbladder
- cholecystopathy (chole/cyst/o/path/y)—any disease of the gallbladder
- cholecystogastric (chole/cyst/o/gastr/ic)—pertaining to the gallbladder and stomach
- cholecystenteric (chole/cyst/enter/ic)—pertaining to the gallbladder and intestines

chondr-   cartilage; gristle; a firm elastic tissue serving principally to connect body parts

Important locations of cartilage are in joints, such as between the vertebrae of the spine, in the connections between the ribs and the breastbone (sternum) and in the connections of the ribs with each other.

Examples:

- chondral (chondr/al)—pertaining to cartilage; "of the cartilage"
- chondroma (chondr/oma)—a tumor composed of cartilage
- chondropathology (chondr/o/path/ology)—the study of diseases of the cartilage
- chondrotomy (chondr/otomy)—the surgical cutting of cartilage
- chondritis (chondr/itis)— inflammation of cartilage
- chondrectomy (chondr/ectomy)—surgical excision (removal of cartilage)
- chondrodermatitis (chondr/o/dermat/itis)—inflammation involving both cartilage and skin

crani-   skull; the cranium; the bone structure (skeleton) of the head

Both *crani-* (the root) and cranium (the name) are used to variously denote three different structures, all of which refer to bones of the head:

1. All the bones of the head
2. All the bones of the head except the lower jaw (the mandible)
3. The brain case or brain enclosure; that is, all the bones surrounding the brain, known as the 8 cranial bones. This usage excludes the lower jaw and the other bones forming the face, such as the bones of the nose, the cheek bones, the upper jawbone and the bones underlying the roof of the mouth

Examples:

- cranial (crani/al)—pertaining to the skull or cranium; as a directional term, pertaining to the end or portion of an organ or other body part that is nearer to the head
- craniectomy (crani/ectomy)—excision (surgical removal) of a part of the skull
- craniomalacia (crani/o/malacia)—abnormal softening of the skull
- craniopathy (crani/o/path/y)—any disease of the skull
- craniopuncture (crani/o/puncture)—puncture of the skull to search for cranial disease

cyan-   blue; generally a deep or dark blue

Examples:

- cyanic (cyan/ic)—pertaining to the color blue
- cyanoderma (cyan/o/derm/a)—a bluish discoloration of the skin

☞   **Note:** The root *cyan-* also applies to a group of chemical substances. (Cyanide, you may recall, is a poison frequently employed by writers of mystery fiction.) Apart from this chemical designation, most medical terms in which *cyan-* appears have to do with an appearance of blueness (usually abnormal) in a body part, particularly the skin and mucous membranes, usually due to a reduction of the red coloring matter of the blood. The medical words for this condition are cyanosis (cyan/osis) and cyanopathy (cyan/o/path/y).

cyst   sac containing fluid; bladder; a pouch or baglike structure or organ

The spelling "sac" is not a typographical error for "sack." "Sac" is the medical term which is practically identical in meaning with our ordinary meaning of "sack" in the sense of a bag for holding things. The major difference: "sacks" are usually large; "sacs" may be, and usually are, small.

A "bladder" is used in medical terms to denote a sac composed of membrane, usually serving as a receptacle for secretions, principally urine (urinary bladder) and bile or gall (gallbladder or cholecyst-). When "bladder" is used with no other description, it means the urinary bladder.

✳ "Cyst" used as a word ("a cyst") usually means an abnormal sac containing liquid or semisolid materials; a tumor containing the products of inflammation such as pus.

"*cyst-*" as a word element usually denotes a body structure of saclike form; a bladder.

Examples:
- cystalgia (cyst/algia)—pain in the urinary bladder
- cholecystalgia (chole/cyst/algia)—pain in the gallbladder
- cystospasm (cyst/o/spasm)—spasm of the urinary bladder
- endocystitis (end/o/cyst/itis)—inflammation of the membrane lining the urinary bladder

☞ **Note:** *Cyst-* may be used to denote both an abnormal sac containing fluid and the normal saclike structures of the body such as the urinary bladder and the gallbladder.

Examples:
- cystic (cyst/ic)—pertaining to a cyst; pertaining to the urinary bladder or the gallbladder
- cystectomy (cyst/ectomy)—excision of a cyst; excision of the urinary bladder

end-   inside; within; inner (sometimes seen in the form *ent-*)

ium ⟩ lining
itis ⟩
osis ⟩

This prefix is generally used to indicate (in the sense of "pointing to") the inside of some body part.

It may name the inner lining (usually a membrane) using the form end/o/____/ium.

Examples:
- endangium (end/angi/um)—the inner lining of a blood vessel
- endocardium (end/o/cardi/um)—the inner lining membrane of the heart

It may also refer to ("pertaining to") the inside of a structure or organ in the form end/o/_____/al, such as:
- endarterial (end/arter/i/al)—within an artery
- endocardial (end/o/cardi/al)—situated or occurring within the heart; pertaining to the endocardium (see above)

It may also indicate a condition through the forms end/o/_____/itis, end/o/_____/osis:

- endangiitis (end/angi/itis)—inflammation of the inner lining of a blood vessel (endangium—see above)
- endocarditis (end/o/card/itis)—inflammation of the lining of the heart (endocardium—see above)
- entostosis (ent/ost/osis)—an abnormal bony growth within the hollow interior of a bone

---

hem(at)-   blood; the fluid that circulates in the heart (cardi-) and blood vessels (hemangi-) carrying nourishment and oxygen to the body cells

---

☞   **Note:** You are encountering here two principles or rules which also occur in roots in subsequent lessons:

1. If a root ends with the letter "m," it may also have the form *"-mat-."* This appears in many common English words:

- syste*m*/syste*mat*ic
- dra*m*(a)/dra*mat*ic
- sche*m*(e)/sche*mat*ic
- sympto*m*/sympto*mat*ic
- trau*m*(a)/trau*mat*ic

Examples of the element *hem-* that ends with the letter "m" being used in the form he*mat:*

- he*mat*ology—the study of the blood
- he*mat*ologist—a specialist in the study of blood
- he*mat*ic—pertaining to the blood
- he*mat*oma—a tumor containing blood

2. If a root begins with the letter "h," it will retain the "h" if it begins a word; however, if the root is preceded by some other element, the "h" will usually be dropped.

Examples of the letter "h" being **retained** when the element *hem-* appears at the beginning of a medical term:

- *hem*angioma—a tumor made up of blood vessels
- *hem*ic—pertaining to the blood
- *hem*atology—the study of the blood

Examples of the letter "h" being **dropped** when the element *hem-* appears *within* the medical term:

- cyan*em*ia—a bluish condition of the blood
- hyper*em*ia—an excess (more than normal) amount of blood in a body part

☞   **Note:** The form *-emia* appears often within medical terms. It means "condition of the blood." Please note that *-emia* is actually *hemia* with the letter "h" dropped.

hemi-   half; half of; relating to or affecting a half or one side; sometimes "a part of"

Examples:
- hemialgia (hemi/algia)—pain affecting one side of the body only
- hemicrania (hemi/cran/ia)—pain or aching on one side of the head
- hemihepatectomy (hemi/hepat/ectomy)—surgical removal of part of the liver
- hemisection (hemi/section)—a division into two sections; a cutting in which the part cut is divided into two sections
- hemispasm (hemi/spasm)—a spasm affecting one side of the body only
- hemigastrectomy (hemi/gastr/ectomy)—excision of one half of the stomach

hyper-   above, more than normal; excessive; opposite of *hypo-* (underneath or deficient)

Although the prefix may be used in the sense of "located above," the sense of the meaning in medical terms is almost always that of "excessive" or "more than normal."

Examples:
- hyperalgia (hyper/algia)—excessive pain; excessive sensitivity to pain
- hyperemia (hyper/em/ia)—an excess of blood in a body part
- hypernormal (hyper/normal)—in excess of that which is normal
- hyperpsychosis (hyper/psych/osis)—an exaggeration of mental (mind) activity, especially as exhibited by abnormal rapidity of the flow of thought
- hyperostosis (hyper/ost/osis)—excessive formation of bone tissue, especially in the skin
- hypertension (hyper/tension)—excessive tension; more than normal blood pressure; "high blood pressure"

hypo-   under; beneath; deficient; less than normal; underneath or below in space; opposite of *hyper-*

Unlike its opposite *hyper-*, the prefix *hypo-* carries two senses of "under" in its medical applications. One is the sense of "deficient," "less than normal":
- hypoadenia (hypo/aden/ia)—abnormally diminished glandular activity (also hypo/glandular)
- hypohepatia (hypo/hepat/ia)—deficient functioning of the liver
- hypotension (hypo/tension)—diminished tension; lowered blood pressure; "low blood pressure"

A number of medical words containing *hypo-* carry the sense "underneath or beneath in space":
- hypodermic (hypo/derm/ic)—underneath the skin; a hypodermic needle is inserted below the skin
- hypogastrium (hypo/gastr/ium)—the region of the lowest part of the abdomen

hyster- uterus; womb; hollow, muscular organ in the female in which the egg (ovum) is deposited and in which the unborn young is developed and nourished

Examples:
- hysteralgia (hyster/algia)—pain in the uterus
- hysterectomy (hyster/ectomy)—surgical removal (excision) of the uterus
- hysterocervicotomy (hyster/o/cervic/otomy)—incision of the neck of the uterus and the lower part of the uterus to relieve difficult labor
- hysterology (hyster/ology)—study of the uterus

lip- fat; fatty; fatty tissue

Examples:
- lipoid (lip/oid)—resembling fat; fatlike
- lip- denotes the oily or greasy substance that occurs in many parts of the body:

  lipocardiac (lip/o/cardi/ac)—a fatty heart
  lipemia (lip/em/ia)—abnormal fat in the blood
  lipoarthritis (lip/o/arthr/itis)—inflammation of the fatty tissue of a joint

Many tumors consist of fatty substances (lip/oma), or the tumor may contain other substances in addition to fat:
- fibrolipoma (fibr/o/lip/oma)—a tumor containing fiberlike (threadlike) structure and fat
- myolipoma (my/o/lip/oma)—a tumor made up of muscle and fat elements

lith- stone; a mass of extremely hard material; a calculus (an abnormal hardening of body substances or chemicals, particularly mineral salts)

Examples:
- lithic (lith/ic)—pertaining to a stone or stones
- -lithia, -lithiasis (-lith/iasis)—the abnormal forming of stony material

Abnormal formations of stony material may occur throughout the body. Familiar terms may be gallstones (chole/lith-), kidney stones (nephr/o/lith-). The condition *-lithia* or *-lithiasis* (also called concretion) may occur, for example, in the joints (arthr/o/ lith/iasis), the urinary bladder (cyst/o/lith/iasis) and the appendix (append/ic/ul/ar lith/iasis).

-lysis loosening; set free; destruction; release; breaking down; decomposition; freeing; dissolving

Lysis is a word meaning destruction; decomposition as of a chemical compound; loosening, as of an organ from adhesions (an abnormal "sticking together" of adjoining parts of the body).

Lysis most frequently occurs in medical terms as the suffix *-lysis*:
- litholysis (lith/o/lysis)—the dissolving of stones in the bladder, that is, the urinary bladder
- hemolysis (hem/o/lysis)—the breaking down and dissolving of red blood cells
- gastrolysis (gastr/o/lysis)—the operation of loosening the stomach from adhesions
- autolysis (auto/lysis)—the destruction of body tissues or cells due to internal causes

my- muscle; body organs consisting of bundles of cells or fibers that can be contracted and expanded to produce bodily movement.

Examples:
- myoma, -myoma (my/oma, -my/oma)—a tumor made up of muscular elements
- angiomyoma (angi/o/my/oma)—a tumor consisting of blood and muscle elements; specifically a tumor consisting of a coil of blood vessels surrounded by a network of muscular fibers

Just as *hem-* occasionally appears in a medical term as *hemat-*, the element *oma-* occasionally appears as *omat-*:
- myomatectomy (my/omat/ectomy)—surgical removal of a muscle tumor (a myoma)

-oid like; resembling; having the form or shape of

Used widely in medical terms to name body parts, tissues or fluids by attaching the suffix to other body parts, tissues or fluids that the named thing resembles. Descriptive names for tumors as alternatives to -oma suffixed words include:
- adenoid (aden/oid) tumor—a tumor consisting of glandular or glandlike material; an adenoma
- dermoid (derm/oid) tumor—a tumor containing skinlike elements
- fibroid (fibr/oid) tumor—a tumor containing fiberlike structures; a fibroma

A cystoid (cyst/oid) is like a cyst in being a soft mass but lacks an enclosing capsule which is present in a true cyst.
- lipoid (lip/oid)—like or resembling fat
- myoid (my/oid)—like or resembling a muscle

ophthalm- the eye or eyes
opt- seeing; vision; light

Examples:
- ophthalmologist (ophthalm/ologist)—a specialist in the study of the eyes
- ophthalmic (ophthalm/ic)—pertaining to the eye or eyes

- ophthalmolith (ophthalm/o/lith)—a stonelike substance in the eye
- ophthalmalacia (ophthal/malacia)—abnormal softening of the eye; note that the "m" of ophthalm- has been dropped because of the presence of the initial "m" of malacia
- optic, optical (opt/ic, opt/ic/al)—pertaining to the eye; pertaining to vision or sight; by extension, also pertaining to light

> ☞ **Note:** Technically, optic is used to refer to (pertain to) the eye and optical to refer to (pertain to) sight.

As you probably know, particularly if you have needed eyeglasses, there are three different names for people dealing with eyeglasses: ophthalmologist, optometrist and optician.

An ophthalmologist (opthalm/ologist) is a physician, a doctor of medicine, specializing in the treatment of diseases of the eye.

An optometrist (opt/o/metr/ist) is a doctor of optometry clinically trained and licensed to treat visual defects with corrective lenses and other methods that do not require license as a physician .

An optician (opt/ic/ian) is one who prepares lenses in accordance with the prescription of the ophthalmologist or the optometrist and supplies eyeglasses.

⚹ ost-   bone; bone tissue

This element may appear in the forms ost-, oste-, oss-, ossi-, osse-.

ost- and *oste-* are the roots in words dealing with disease conditions and the therapeutic procedures to correct such disease conditions:

- ostalgia (ost/algia) also ostealgia (oste/algia)—pain in the bone or bones
- osteoma (oste/oma)—a tumor composed of bone tissue
- osteopathy (oste/o/path/y)—any disease of the bone; a name for a system of healing which originally relied on manipulation of bones to diagnose and correct disease but which now uses generally accepted physical, medicinal and surgical methods of diagnosis and treatment
- osteopath (oste/o/path)—one who practices osteopathy
- osteoarthropathy (oste/o/arthr/o/path/y)—any disease of the bones and joints
- ⚹ ossicle (oss/i/cle)—a small bone, particularly the small bones of the ear

⚹*oss-, ossi-, osse-* are used mostly in the naming of anatomical parts involving bone and normal biological processes involving bone or bone tissue:

Examples:
- osseous (osse/ous)—of the nature or quality of bone or bone tissue; bony
- osteal (oste/al)—of the nature or quality of bone or bone tissue; bony

-ostomy   to create an opening; to provide a new opening; a surgical opening into—; creation of a "mouth"

The suffix stem *-ostomy* denotes a surgical operation in which an artificial opening is made into an organ or structure (enter/ostomy, gastr/ostomy, chole/cyst/ostomy, arthr/ostomy, etc.) for the purposes of drainage or the discharge of body fluids or waste.

-ostomy is also used to denote the creation of a new opening or passage between two or more functionally related organs:

- gastroenterostomy (gastr/o/enter/ostomy)—surgical creation of an artificial passage between the stomach and the intestines
- enterocholecystostomy (enter/o/chole/cyst/ostomy)—surgical creation of an artificial passage between the intestine and the gallbladder
- hepaticocholangiocholecystenterostomy (hepat/ic/o/chol/angi/o/chole/ cyst/enter/ostomy)—surgical creation of an artificial passage between the gallbladder and a liver duct and between the intestine and the gallbladder

The root element in the suffix -ostomy is *stom-* which means "mouth." Since the most prominent of the body openings is the mouth of the face through which we ingest food and through which we speak, the idea of the mouth as a designation for opening was adopted:

- stom-, stomat- a mouth; the mouth; a mouthlike opening
- stomal, stomatal (stom/al, stomat/al)—pertaining to a mouth; pertaining to the mouth
- stoma-, -stoma (stom/a-, -stom/a)—the name for an opening, a mouth, the mouth

Please observe the relationship between *stom-* and *-ostomy* in that "to create a new opening" is to create a mouth or opening.

---

para-   beside; by the side; at the side of; to one side; side by side; beyond
Also, wrong; faulty; disordered

Examples:
- paramedical (para/medic/al)—"side by side with medicine"; having some connection or being related to the practice of medicine, such as the paramedical services of physical, occupational and speech therapists. A "paramedic" or a "paramedical" is one who has been trained in limited medical skills to assist physicians, that is one who works "side by side with a physician."
- paracystitis (para/cyst/itis)—inflammation of the tissues around the bladder (the urinary bladder)
- parosteal (par/oste/al)—"pertaining to the side of the bone"; the outer surface of the membrane covering a bone
- paralysis (para/lysis)—"faulty loosening"; the loss, in a part of the body, of the power of movement

proct- "anus"; the last part of the digestive tube, measuring about 18 centimeters (7 inches) in length, through which the solid waste products remaining after digestion are expelled from the body

☞ **Important Note:** The Dean Vaughn Total Retention System™ has deliberately chosen to use "anus" as the meaning for the element *proct-* in the audiovisual presentation. This was done in order that you might first get a clearer idea of the area of the body to which the element *proct-* applies. We now need to develop the sense in which the element is used to form medical words.

The end of the digestive tube, digestive tract, alimentary tract or canal as it may be called, technically consists of three parts:

1. the anus (an/us)—the opening through which solid waste matter (feces) is expelled
2. the anal (an/al) canal—approximately 4 centimeters (one and one-half inches) long through which waste matter is conducted for expulsion through the anus
3. the rectum (rect/um)—approximately 13 centimeters (five inches) long that serves as a storage pouch for waste material awaiting expulsion

The word rectal (rect/al)—pertains to the rectum, anal canal, and anus

Technically (that is, in precise anatomical descriptions) the element *proct-* is restricted to words dealing with the rectum (the storage pouch). However, medical usage has broadened the application of the element to include, in many applications, the anus, the anal canal and the rectum in its entirety. For example:

- proctology (proct/ology)—branch of medicine dealing with the anus, the anal canal and the rectum
- proctologist (proct/ologist)—a physician skilled in proctology
- proctoplasty (proct/o/plast/y)—the plastic surgery (surgical repair) of the anus and/or the anal canal and/or the rectum

psycho- mind; mental processes; the processes of thought, judgment, and emotion

The element *psych-* should not be confused with the element *cerebr-* (Lesson 1). The brain (*cerebr-*) is a mass of tissue in the cranium (the head, the brain case). *Psych-* (mind) is used to express the behavior resulting from physical processes taking place in the brain (*cerebr-*):

- psychic (psych/ic)—pertaining to the mind
- psyche (psych/e)—the mind

In Lesson 1 we learned the use of *-ology* and *-ologist* and applied these suffixes to the body parts of Lesson 1. We can also derive from Lesson 2 such branches of medical knowledge as:

- hematology (hemat/ology)—dealing with blood and blood-forming tissues
- ophthalmology (ophthalm/ology)—dealing with the eye and its diseases
- proctology (proct/ology)—dealing with the anus, the anal canal and the rectum

Similarly, we can derive hematologist, ophthalmologist and proctologist as names for the physicians skilled in these branches.

You might logically conclude that psychology would name the branch of medical knowledge dealing with the mind and that the word psychologist would designate the physician skilled in the mind and its disease. It is true that psychology is a name for "knowledge of the mind" and that a psychologist is a "knower of the mind." There are psychologists who do diagnose and treat mental disorders. Such a practitioner is named "clinical psychologist" ("clinical" deriving from *clinic-* meaning the direct observation and treatment of patients as distinguished from experimental or laboratory study + -al, "pertaining to"). The field is clinical psychology.

In contrast, the field of medicine dealing with the mind is psychiatry. The root *iatr-* means "healing" and is widely used in medical terms. A psych*iatr*ist is "one who heals the mind."

To summarize:

an -*ologist* is always a "knower" and may be a physician, "a healer"

an "-*iatrist* is always a physician, "a healer"

a *clinical psychologist* may provide treatment for mental disorders but is limited by his license or by the laws and regulations governing medical practice as such laws apply to other than physicians

a *psychiatrist* is "a healer of the mind," a physician and is limited only by the laws and regulations governing physicians

To round out our discussion of "knowledge of," "knowers of" and "healers of" the psyche (mind), you should know that psychoanalysis is a specialized field for investigating mental processes and treating certain mental disorders. Very briefly, the technique assumes that such mental disorders are the result of experiences which have been buried in the mind and that by bringing them into awareness (consciousness) the disorders may be cured or alleviated. You know the meaning of *psych-* and -*lysis*. The prefix *ana-* has a meaning "back or backward." Literally, psychoanalysis means "a state (or condition) of loosening the mind backwards." A psychoanalyst is "one who practices psychoanalysis." A psychoanalyst may or may not be a physician.

| *-scop-* | observe; look; reveal |

The addition of the ending -*e* which carries a meaning "instrument for" forms the suffix stem -scope (-scop/e) meaning "instrument for observing." The stem appears in words with which you are familiar. For example:

- telescope (tele/scop/e)—an instrument for observing distant things (the root *tele-* means "distant")
- microscope (micr/o/scop/e)—an instrument for observing small things (the prefix *micr-*, which will be discussed in Lesson 9, means "small")

This suffix is frequently used in the names of medical instruments:

- stethoscope (steth/o/scop/e)—literally, "an instrument for observing the chest" (*steth-* is a root meaning "chest"); a hearing instrument applied to the chest, back and abdomen to listen to the sounds made by the internal organs such as the heart, lungs, etc., in order to determine their conditions

Lesson 2—Element Recognition

Separate the word terminals, elements, and connecting vowels, of the following medical terms from right to left by inserting a slash mark (/) between them.

Example: heminephrectomy—hemi/nephr/ectomy

gastralgia

craniocerebral

endochondral

hemicraniosis

lipoid

hypercholia

cystolithectomy

cholelith

hypo▮emia

hysteroscopy

cystostomy

paraproctitis

angiolysis

cervicoplasty

chondrodermatitis

cyanosis

hematologist

osteoarthropathy

psychopathology

lipochondroma

myoid

lithocystotomy

ophthalmomyotomy

proctoscopy

nephralgia

crani/otomy

end/angi/itis
inflammation within the vessel *linning*

hyperadenosis

cystectomy

cholecystitis

hypoliposis

rhinoscopy

hysterolysis

parahepatic

chondrolysis

cervicitis

hematoma

osteolipochondroma

lipoarthritis

lithoscope

ophthalmomyitis

proctospasm

Lesson 2—Interpretation Exercise

Complete the following statements by printing the meanings of the elements that make up the medical term in the proper blanks. (Remember, most medical terms are interpreted from right to left.)

2-1.   The term myalgia (my/algia) denotes _____ in a _____.

2-2.   Cervicitis (cervic/itis) is an _____ of the _____ of the uterus

2-3.   A cholecystectomy (chole/cyst/ectomy) is the surgical_____of the _____.

2-4.   The term chondral (chondr/al) denotes pertaining to or of the _____.

2-5.   A craniopunture (crani/o/puncture) is the surgical _____ of the _____.

2-6.   The term cyanoderma (cyan/o/derm/a) pertains to a _____ discoloration of the _____.

2-7.   Cystalgia (cyst/algia) denotes _____ in the _____.

2-8.   Endocardial (end/o/cardi/al) denotes pertaining to _____ the _____.

2-9.   The term hemic (hem/ic) means pertaining to or of the _____.

2-10.   A hemihepatectomy (hemi/hepat/ectomy) is the surgical _____ of _____ the _____.

2-11.   Hyperalgia (hyper/algia) denotes _____ _____.

2-12.   The term hypohepatia (hypo/hepat/ia) pertains to_____ functioning of the_____ .

2-13.   A hysterectomy (hyster/ectomy) is the surgical _____ of the _____.

2-14. A myolipoma (my/o/lip/oma)is a _____ made up of _____
and _____.

2-15. Hepatomegaly (hepat/o/megal/y) denotes an _____ of
the _____.

2-16. The term lithic (lith/ic) means pertaining to a _____.

2-17. An angiomyoma (angi/o/my/oma) is a _____ comprised of blood
_____ and _____.

2-18. The term cystoid (cyst/oid) means _____ a cyst.

2-19. An ophthalmologist (ophthalm/ologist) is a specialist in the _____ of
the _____.

2-20. The term osteoarthropathy (oste/o/arthr/o/path/y) refers to any _____ of the
_____ and _____.

2-21. A gastroenterostomy (gastr/o/enter/ostomy) is the surgical creation of an_____
between the _____ and the _____.

2-22. Paracystitis (para/cyst/itis) is an inflammation of the tissues _____ the
urinary _____.

2-23. Proctoplasty (procto/plast/y) is the surgical _____ of the _____.

2-24. The term psychic (psych/ic) denotes pertaining to or of the _____.

2-25. The term scope (scop/e) denotes an instrument for _____.

Lesson 3

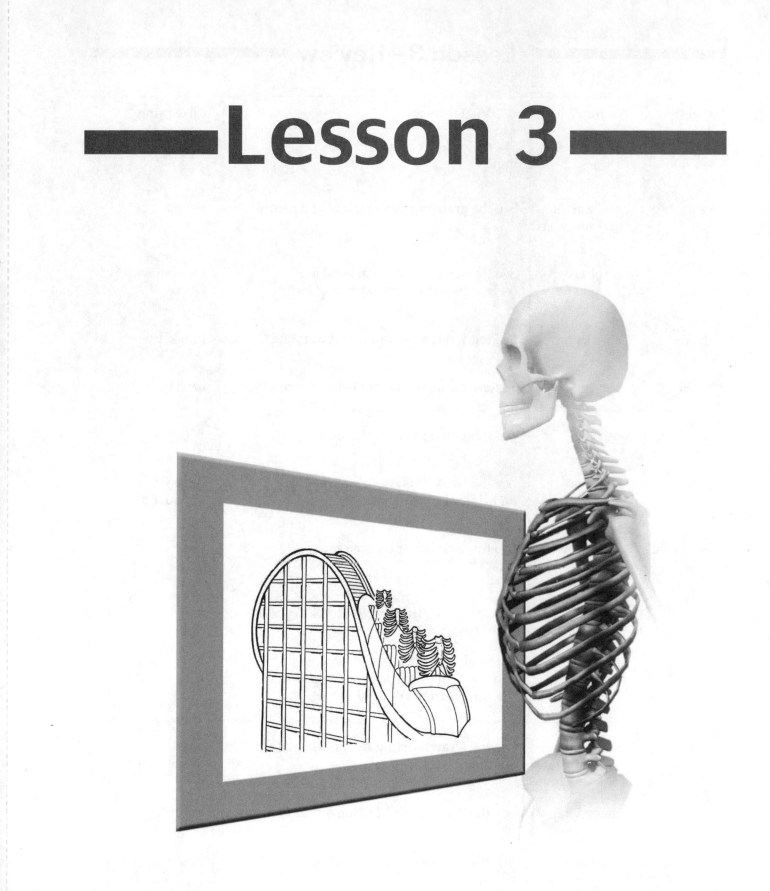

Element	Audionym	Visual Image	Meaning
cost-	coaster	See the roller **coast**er with **rib**s riding in it!	rib
-gram	graham (graham cracker)	See the **gra**ham cracker made of a **record**!	record
acro-	acrobat	See the **acro**bat with arms and legs (extremities) that are **extrem**ely long!	extremities
rhexis	wrecks	See the **wrecks break**ing and **burst**ing!	break, burst
carcin-	car sign	See the **car sign** made of **can**ned **cere**al!	cancer
-penia	pen	See the **pen decreas**ing its ink!	decrease
gen-	Genesis	See the Book of **Gen**esis producing an **original production**!	original, production
burso-	purse sew	See the girl with the **purse sew**ing a **sack**!	sac
retr(o)-	retreat	See the men **retre**ating riding **backwards** on horses!	backwards
trip-	trip	See the man preparing for a **trip, rub**bing the car, creating **friction**!	rub, friction
strept-	strap	See the **strap twist**ing on the woman's shoulder!	twist
-desis	thesis	See the **thesis** with **binding** around it!	binding
mani-	maniac	See the **mani**ac reading **Mad** magazine!	madness

Element	Audionym	Visual Image	Meaning
glosso-	glossy	See the **gloss**y furniture with **tongue**s sticking out of it!	tongue
-trophy	trophy	See the **trophy** that turns into a housing **development**!	development
supra-	soup	See the **soup above** the bowl!	above
-ptosis	toe sis	See "**toe sis**" (the sister with the very big toe) **falling** everywhere she goes!	falling
-dyn-	dinner	See the **din**ner being served through the window**pane**!	pain
mast-	mast	See the **mast** of the ship with a gigantic **breast**plate on it!	breast
-rrhaphy	raffle	See the **raffle** with a suit bursting out of it that has **suture**s all over it!	suture
dent-	dentist	See the **dent**ist with gigantic **teeth**!	teeth
cephal-	sieve fall	See the **sieve fall**ing with a **head** in it!	head
auto-	auto	See the **auto** that can drive it**self**!	self
epi-	a pea	See **a pea** with other peas **upon** it!	upon
hydro-	hydrant	See the **hydr**ant with **water** gushing out of it!	water

Print the audionym and meaning of the elements in the proper blanks:

Element	Audionym	Meaning
cost-	coaster	rib
-gram	grahm cracker	record
acro-	acrobat	extremities
-rhexis	wrecks	break, burst
carcin-	car sign	cancer
-penia	pen	decrease
gen-	genesis	original production
burso-	purse/sew	sac
retr(o)-	retreat	backwards
trip-	trip	rub, friction
strept-	stripped	twist
-desis	thesis	binding
mani-	maniac	madness
glosso-	glossy	tongue
-trophy	trophy	development
supra-	soup	above
-ptosis	toe sis	falling
dyn-	dinner	pain
mast-	mast	breast
-rrhaphy	raffle	suture
dent-	dentist	teeth
cephal-	sieve fall	head
auto-	auto	self
epi-	a pea	upon
hydro-	hydrant	water

Lesson 3

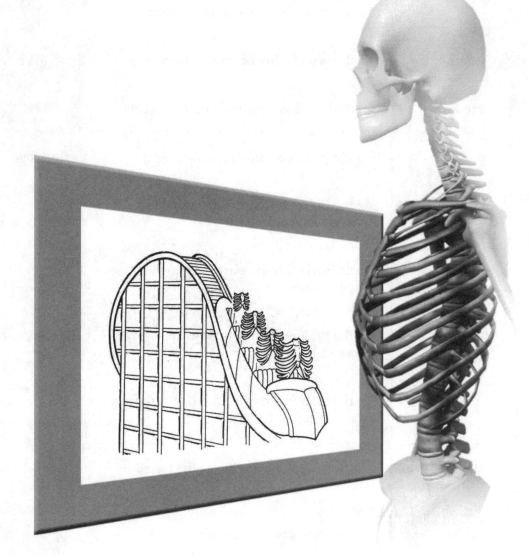

Element	Audionym	Visual Image	Meaning
cost-	coaster	See the roller **coast**er with **rib**s riding in it!	rib
-gram	graham (graham cracker)	See the **gra**ham cracker made of a **record**!	record
acro-	acrobat	See the **acro**bat with arms and legs (extremities) that are **extrem**ely long!	extremities
rhexis	wrecks	See the **wrecks** brea**k**ing and **burst**ing!	break, burst
carcin-	car sign	See the **car sign** made of **can**ned **cer**eal!	cancer
-penia	pen	See the **pen decreas**ing its ink!	decrease
gen-	Genesis	See the Book of **Gen**esis producing an **original production**!	original, production
burso-	purse sew	See the girl with the **purse sew**ing a **sac**k!	sac
retr(o)-	retreat	See the men **retr**eating riding **backwards** on horses!	backwards
trip-	trip	See the man preparing for a **trip, rub**bing the car, creating **friction**!	rub, friction
strept-	stripped	See the lady **strip**ping to do the **twist**!	twist
-desis	thesis	See the **thesis** with **binding** around it!	binding
mani-	maniac	See the **mani**ac reading **Mad** magazine!	madness

Lesson 3—Review

Element	Audionym	Visual Image	Meaning
glosso-	glossy	See the **gloss**y furniture with **tongue**s sticking out of it!	tongue
-trophy	trophy	See the **trophy** that turns into a housing **development**!	development
supra-	soup	See the **soup above** the empty bowl!	above
-ptosis	toe sis	See "**toe sis**" (the sister with the very big toe) **falling** everywhere she goes!	falling
-dyn-	dinner	See the **din**ner being served through the window**pane**!	pain
mast-	mast	See the **mast** of the ship with a **breast** on it!	breast
-rrhaphy	raffle	See the **raffle** with a suit bursting out of it that has **suture**s all over it!	suture
dent-	dentist	See the **dent**ist with very very long **teeth**!	teeth
cephal-	sieve fall	See the **sieve fal**ling with a **head** in it!	head
auto-	auto	See the **auto** that can drive it**self**!	self
epi-	a pea	See **a pea** with other peas **upon** it!	upon
hydro-	hydrant	See the **hydr**ant with **water** gushing out of it!	water

Substitute this page for use with all previous program editions.

Lesson 3—Worksheet

Print the audionym and meaning of the elements in the proper blanks:

Element	Audionym	Meaning
cost-	_____	_____
-gram	_____	_____
acro-	_____	_____
-rhexis	_____	_____
carcin-	_____	_____
-penia	_____	_____
gen-	_____	_____
burso-	_____	_____
retr(o)-	_____	_____
trip-	_____	_____
strept-	_____	_____
-desis	_____	_____
mani-	_____	_____
glosso-	_____	_____
-trophy	_____	_____
supra-	_____	_____
-ptosis	_____	_____
dyn-	_____	_____
mast-	_____	_____
-rrhaphy	_____	_____
dent-	_____	_____
cephal-	_____	_____
auto-	_____	_____
epi-	_____	_____
hydro-	_____	_____

-ate   to perform; to put into action; to bring about

Examples:
- intoxicate (intoxic/ate)—to bring about a state of drunkenness or intoxication
- fixate (fix/ate)—to fix
- vacate (vac/ate)—to make vacant

-ac ✳   affected by, having; frequently, one who is affected by (Note: In Lesson 1 an additional meaning of **-ac** meaning "pertaining to" was presented.)

Example:
- maniac (mani/ac)—a wildly or violently insane person

-ad ✳   toward, in the direction of

Examples:
- cephalad (cephal/ad)—toward or in the direction of the head
- retrad (retr/ad)—toward the back

This terminal is rare in that it also can be used as a prefix with the same meaning:
- adnerval (ad/nerval)—toward a nerve
- adaxial (ad/axial)—toward an axis

-form   having the same form; shaped like; resembling

Examples:
- dentiform (denti/form)—shaped like a tooth
- uniform (uni/form)—the element **uni-** means one; therefore, a uniform means "all of one shape"; "all of one form"

-ion   action; condition resulting from action

Examples:
- incision (incis/ion)—the act or result of cutting into
- action (act/ion)—the result of acting

-ior	roughly meaning "more toward"

This terminal is called a "comparative" by the dictionaries and indicates "a higher degree." It corresponds to many common English words ending in *-er*.

Examples:

- super/ior   high/er   more above
- inter/ior   inn/er   more toward the inside
- exter/ior   out/er   more toward the outside

-or	action; result; that which does something or has some particular function

Examples:

- elevator (elevat/or)—that which elevates or raises
- flexor (flex/or)—that which flexes or bends
- incisor (incis/or)—that which incises or cuts into

-ous	full of; abounding in; having

Examples:

- fam/ous, danger/ous, poison/ous, joy/ous, nerv/ous, osse/ous

-ure	result of an action; means of an action; device

Examples:

- exposure (expos/ure)—result of being exposed
- pressure (press/ure)—the result of pressing
- legislature (legislat/ure)—a means or device for legislating, that is, passing laws
- denture (dent/ure)—a device for replacing teeth
- pleasure (pleas/ure)—the result of being pleased

Lesson 3—Reading Assignment

acro- extremities; tip; end; a top or peak; extremity of the body; outermost portion

Extremities (singular extremity) is a general word in medical terminology used to designate an outmost or ending portion of an organ or part; a part located away from the center of the body or away from a point of attachment.

"The extremities" in skeletal anatomy (bone parts and structures) technically include the bones of the shoulders and hips, the bones of the wrists and ankles, the bones of the hands and feet. This is the meaning in Gray's Anatomy which is the most widely used text in human anatomy.

Or, the use of "extremity" or "extremities" may refer to each or all:

1. toes and fingers
2. feet and hands
3. wrists and ankles
4. arms and legs

Note that whatever the reference, "extremity" or *acro-* always includes the farthest ends and all parts leading to the farthest end.

Examples:
- acral (acr/al)—pertaining to the extremities or tip; affecting the extremities
- acrodermatitis (acro/dermat/itis)—inflammation of the skin of the hands and feet
- acromegaly (acro/megal/y)—enlargement of the extremities of the skeleton— the fingers, toes, nose and jaws (also megal/acr/ia)
- acrocyanosis (acro/cyan/osis)—blueness of the extremities (fingers, toes, wrists, ankles)

auto- self/same one; self-caused; occurring within one's own body

Examples:
- autocystoplasty (auto/cyst/o/plast/y)—a plastic operation on the bladder with grafts from the patient's own body
- autohemotherapy (auto/hemo/therap/y)—treatment by injection of the patient's own blood (also auto/infusion)
- autolysis (auto/lysis)—disintegration of tissue due to causes within the patient's own body
- autoplasty (auto/plasty)—the surgical reconstruction of diseased or injured parts by tissue taken from another part of the patient's own body
- autoscope (auto/scop/e)—an instrument for the examination of one's own organs

sac in a joint

burso- sac; any baglike cavity, especially a sac containing lubricating fluid at places of friction in the body

Examples:
- bursa (burs/a)—the bursa are closed sacs that contain fluid and lie between surfaces that glide over each other. They lie between the skin and prominent bones such as those of the elbows, shoulders, knees, knuckles and heels; they also lie between the tendons and the surfaces on which the tendons glide. They serve to reduce friction at these points.
- bursitis (burs/itis)—inflammation of a bursa
- bursopathy (burso/path/y)—any disease of a bursa
- bursolith (burso/lith)—hard, stonelike deposits in a bursa
- bursotomy (burs/otomy)—surgical incision of a bursa

carcin- cancer; a malignant (bad, harmful) new growth

Cancer is the name used to designate a mass of harmful abnormal tissue cells that grow by invading and spreading throughout the body.

Examples:
- carcinous (carcin/ous)—pertaining to cancer; cancerous (also called carcin/omat/ous)
- carcinoma (carcin/oma)—harmful and life-threatening (malignant) growth tending to infiltrate the surrounding tissues
- carcinosis (carcin/osis)—the spreading of cancer throughout the body
- adenocarcinoma (aden/o/carcin/oma)—a carcinous tumor composed of glandlike cells

cephal- head; the head

Examples:
- cephalic (cephal/ic)—pertaining to the head; especially directed toward or situated on or in or near the head
- cephalad (cephal/ad)—toward the head end of the body
- -cephalus (-cephal/us)—a head abnormality of a specific type

An important use of *cephal-* is the formation of the combination *encephal-* (en/cephal-). The prefix *en-* has a meaning "within" and is discussed in Lesson 9. Literally, then, *encephal-* means "within the head." The largest organ within the head is a mass of nerve tissue called the brain. *Encephal-*, therefore, means "brain:"
- encephal- (en/cephal-)—brain
- encephalic (en/cephal/ic)—pertaining to the brain; lying within the brain cavity

So far we have had five elements which may be creating some confusion in your mind (your psyche) and, therefore, ought to be clarified:

1. *crani-* the framework of bone containing the brain; sometimes used to denote the skull (the entire bony framework of the head)

2. *cephal-* the head in its entirety, including the cranium, the brain, the organs of special sense (eyes, ears, etc.)
3. *cerebr-* in its narrowest application, the *cerebrum,* the main part of the brain in which the higher mental processes take place; sometimes used to denote the entire brain; sometimes used to denote mental processes
4. *encephal-* the entire brain, the tissue structure that constitutes the organ of thought and neural coordination
5. *psych-* the mind; mental processes and activities

To summarize:

crani-, cephal- and *encephal-* always refer to anatomical (body) parts

cerebr- mainly refers to anatomical parts; sometimes may be used in words denoting mental processes and activities

psych- always refers to mental processes and activities, never to anatomical parts

---

cost- rib

Examples:
- costal (cost/al)—pertaining to a rib; related to or situated near ribs
- chondrocostal (chondr/o/cost/al)—of or pertaining to the ribs and rib cartilage
- epicostal (epi/cost/al)—situated upon a rib
- costa (cost/a)—a rib
- costae (cost/ae)—the ribs (plural of costa)
- costicervical (cost/i/cervic/al)—pertaining to or connecting the ribs and neck

---

dent- teeth; the teeth; tooth

Examples:
- dental (dent/al)—pertaining to the teeth
- dentist (dent/ist)—one whose profession it is to treat diseases of the teeth and associated tissues and to supply and insert replacements for lost and damaged teeth; also called dental surgeon and doctor of dental surgery (D.D.S.)
- denture (dent/ure)—an entire set of natural or artificial teeth; ordinarily used to designate an artificial replacement for the natural teeth
- dentiform (dent/i/form)—formed or shaped like a tooth

-desis binding, fixation; surgical union, usually by fusion, that is the formation of a stiff joint through removing intervening tissue and permitting the bony parts to grow together

Example:
- arthrodesis (arthr/o/desis)—surgical fusion of a joint

☞   **Note:** *-pexy* is more widely used than *-desis* for surgical fixation

-dyn-/odyn- pain

-dyn- is taught as a shortened form of the element *odyn-* which carries the same meaning of pain as the element *-algia,* discussed in Lesson 2.

Examples:

- odynometer (odyn/o/meter)—an instrument for measuring pain

-odynia (-odyn/ia)—state of pain; condition of pain:
- arthrodynia (arthr/odyn/ia)—arthr/algia; pain in a joint
- myodynia (my/odyn/ia)—my/algia; pain in a muscle
- glossodynia (gloss/odyn/ia)—gloss/algia; pain in the tongue
- odynolysis (odyn/o/lysis)—"loosening of pain"; relief of pain
- acrodynia (acr/odyn/ia)—pain in the extremities

epi- upon, in addition to / on; over; outer (frequently in the sense "covering")

This prefix is used extensively to name tissue structures or regions of the body in relation to other body parts.

Examples:

- epidermis (epi/derm/is)—"outer skin"; the outermost layer of skin; also called epiderm
- epicyst- (epi/cyst-)—"over bladder"; the structures above the bladder
- epigastrium (epi/gastr/ium)—the upper middle region of the abdomen
- epithelium (epi/ thel/ium)—the covering of internal and external surfaces of the body, including the lining of vessels and other small cavities (*thel-* a root having "tissue" as one of its meanings; the root will be discussed more fully in Lesson 11)

gen- origin / production / originate; produce; formation; bring forth; arise in; be the source of; the beginning of

This is an important root having many applications, not only in medicine but in other sciences and common speech. It is used in many words.

Examples:

- gene (gen/e)—the basic producer (generator) of heredity
- genit—form for words relating to the reproductive system and the organs of reproduction
- genital (genit/al)—pertaining to reproduction or to the organs of reproduction (genit/al/ia—organs of reproduction)
- genitoplasty (genit/o/plast/y)—surgical repair on the genital organs

It is in the form of suffix combinations that the root produces (generates) many medical terms.

-gen—that which produces, a producer (generator); that which is produced:
- carcinogen (carcin/o/gen)—"cancer producer"; any cancer producing substance
- allergen (aller/gen)—"allergy producer"
- pathogen (path/o/gen)—"disease producer"

> **Note:** Disease producers contained in and transmitted through blood are called bloodborne pathogens. The human immunodeficiency virus (HIV) which attacks the body's immune system causing the disease known as Acquired Immune Deficiency Syndrome (AIDS) and the hepatitis B virus (HBV) that can severely damage the liver are two major bloodborne pathogens.

- hydrogen (hydro/gen)—"water producer"; the chemical element
- autogen (auto/gen)— "self producer"; produced within the body as opposed to outside sources

-genesis—the process or condition leading to production of:
- carcinogenesis (carcin/o/genesis)—the production of cancer
- hypergenesis (hyper/genesis)—excessive development (excessive production)
- autogenesis (auto/genesis)—"self generation" originating within the body

-genic and -genous (-gen/ic, -gen/ous)—producing; originating; giving rise to:
- endogenous (end/o/gen/ous)—"originating within"; growing from within; originating or developing within the body; arising from causes within the body as opposed to causes outside of the body as, for example, a tissue for grafting which may be taken from the patient's own body (auto/gen/ous)
- carcinogenic, carcinogenous (carcin/o/gen/ic, carcin/o/gen/ous)—producing cancer; pertaining to a carcinogen
- myogenic (my/o/gen/ic)—giving rise to or forming muscle tissue
- myogenous (my/o/gen/ous)—originating in the muscle tissue

| *glosso-* | tongue |

Examples:
- glossal (gloss/al)—pertaining to the tongue
- hypoglossal (hypo/gloss/al)— underneath the tongue
- glossorrhaphy (glosso/rrhaphy)—suture of the tongue
- glossodynia, glossalgia (glosso/dyn/ia, gloss/algia)—pain in the tongue
- glossoscopy (glosso/scop/y)—looking at, observing, examining or inspecting the tongue

-gram   record; write; a record; a writing; a drawing; especially the written record of an instrument

This suffix is used principally in medicine to denote the record that is drawn or written by an instrument. The suffix denoting the instrument is *-graph*.

- cardiogram (cardi/o/gram)—a record made by an instrument (cardi/o/graph) to show the beats of the heart
- myogram *(my/o/gram)*—a record or tracing made by an apparatus (my/o/graph) to record the effects of muscular contraction

Radiograph (radi/o/graph/y)—*(radi-* means "ray" and is more fully discussed in Lesson 8) denotes the act of making records (principally photographs) through the use of rays (principally X-rays)

☞   **Note:** Although, technically, *-gram* denotes the record and *-graph*, the instrument, gradual usage has led to the practice of using *-graph* as well as *-gram* in naming the record. This is particularly the case in radiography where radiograph and radiogram may be used interchangeably to designate the record.

hydro-   ⌒⌒⌒ fluid, particularly the accumulation of fluid in a body part

☞ ✳ **Note:** *hydro-* may also appear as *hidr-* when referring to a sweat gland and as *hygr-* when referring to moisture

Examples:
- hydric (hydr/ic)—pertaining to water
- hidro—form denoting relationship to sweat or a sweat gland
- hidrocystoma (hidro/cyst/oma)—a cyst (pouch, bag) of the sweat gland consisting of retained (that is, "not secreted") sweat
- hydrocyst (hydro/cyst)—a cyst (pouch, bag) filled with water
- hydremia (hydr/em/ia)—a watery state of the blood
- hidrosis (hidr/osis)—any skin disease affecting the sweat glands
- hygro— "moist" or denoting relationship to water or fluids
- hygric (hygr/ic)—pertaining to moisture or fluids
- hygroma (hygr/oma)—a sac, cyst or bursa distended (stretched) with a fluid

mani-   madness; mental disturbance, a state of mind in which there is loss of control over emotional, nervous or mental processes

Examples:
- mania (mani/a)—a phase of mental disorder in which there is loss of control over emotional, nervous, or mental processes
- manic (man/ic)—pertaining to mania; affected with mania
- maniac (mani/ac)—one who is affected with mania
- manic-depressive psychosis (man/ic, psych/osis)—a psychosis (mind disorder) characterized by emotional instability and striking mood swings

- -mania (-mani/a)—a suffix stem used to signify obsessive preoccupation with something:

  - kleptomania (klept/o/mani/a)—(*klept-* means theft or stealing)
  - megalomania (megal/o/mani/a)—"largeness obsession"; delusion of grandeur; unreasonable conviction of one's own extreme greatness, goodness or power

---

mast-   breast; the front part of the chest

☞   **Note:** There is a small bony projection behind the ear called the mastoid (mast/oid) process, so named because its shape resembles that of a breast; *masto-* may be encountered in reference to the mastoid process, but usually with a following element that clearly limits the meaning.

☞   **Note:** Words containing *mastic-* do *not* mean "pertaining to the breast" but are related to mastication (the chewing of food).

Apart from the qualifications regarding the mastoid process and mastication, the element *mast-* may denote the front of the chest (male or female) or one or both of the two masses of tissue forming the milk-secreting glands in the female.

Examples:
- mastitis (mast/itis)—inflammation of the breast or the milk-secreting gland
- mastostomy (mast/ostomy)—incision of the breast to provide an opening for drainage
- mastaden (mast/aden)—the milk-secreting gland in the female
- mastectomy (mast/ectomy)—the surgical removal of a breast or part of a breast

Mamm-, a root applying exclusively to the milk secreting gland, is discussed in Lesson 9.

-penia   decrease; deficiency of; less than; less than usual

Examples:
- hematopenia (hemat/o/penia)—deficiency of blood in the body
- lipopenia (lip/o/penia)—deficiency of lipids (fatlike chemicals such as acids) in the body
- cytopenia (cyt/o/penia)—deficiency of the cellular elements of the body
- leukopenia (leuk/o/penia)—reduction in the number of white blood cells; also called leukocytopenia
- erythropenia (erythr/o/penia)—deficiency in the number of red blood cells; also called erythrocytopenia
- hydropenia (hydro/penia)—deficiency of water in the body

-penic (-pen/ic)—pertaining to a state of deficiency

-ptosis   falling; sagging, drooping, a downward displacement

Ptosis is a medical term meaning the falling or drooping of an organ or body part. It is used most frequently as a suffix.

Examples:
- hepatoptosis (hepat/o/ptosis)—a condition in which the liver is displaced downward from its normal position
- gastroptosis (gastr/o/ptosis)—downward displacement of the stomach
- cystoptosis (cyst/o/ptosis)—downward displacement of the urinary bladder
- hysteroptosis (hyster/o/ptosis)—downward displacement of the uterus (womb)
- blepharoptosis (blephar/o/ptosis)—drooping of upper eyelid

retr(o)-   backwards / back; situated behind; contrary to the usual or natural course

Examples:
- retraction (retr/action)—the act of drawing back
- retractor (retr/actor)—an instrument for drawing back the edges of a wound
- retrocardiac (retro/cardi/ac)—behind the heart
- retronasal (retro/nasal)—behind the nose
- retroversion (retro/version)—the tipping of an entire organ backward (*vers-* is a root meaning turning; -vers/ion is the act or action of turning)

-rrhaphy   (the word rhaphy used as the ending *-raphy* *) suture; suturing; the action of joining together the edges of a rupture, wound, or incision, principally by stitching; the action of repairing or reattaching body parts that have become torn from or separated from their points of attachment.

* *-rrh-:* when the combining form of a root is added in front of another root beginning with *rh-*, a second *-r* is nearly always inserted forming the combination *-rrh-*.

Examples:
- myorrhaphy (my/o/rrhaphy)—a suture or suturing of a muscle
- cardiorrhaphy (cardi/o/rrhaphy)—a suture or suturing of the heart or heart muscle
- proctorrhaphy (proct/o/rrhaphy)—a suture or suturing of the rectum
- nephrorrhaphy (nephr/o/rrhaphy)—the sewing in position of a displaced kidney

-rrhexis   a word meaning a bursting; a rupture; a forcible tearing apart. Used often as a word ending. Its meaning can range from a bursting or splitting of a major organ to the minor splitting of a fingernail.

Examples:
- cardiorrhexis (cardi/o/rrhexis)—rupture of the heart
- angiorrhexis (angi/o/rrhexis)—rupture of a blood vessel

- hysterorrhexis (hyster/o/rrhexis)—rupture of the uterus
- onychorrhexis (onych/o/rrhexis)—splitting and brittleness of the fingernail or toenail

Another form, *rhagad-*, also has a similar meaning of a split; crack; fissure:
- rhagades (rhagad/es)—fissures or cracks in the skin
- rhagadiform (rhagad/i/form)—in the form of fissures; fissured; containing cracks

strept-	twist / twisted

This element is most familiarly used in the expression "strep throat" ("strept throat") as an abbreviation for "streptococcal infection of the throat."

Example:
- streptococcus (strept/o/coccus)—name of an infectious microorganism so called because of its twisted form

supra-	above; over / higher than; located or situated on the upper side of; directly above

Examples:
- supracerebral (supra/cerebr/al)—over or on the surface of the cerebrum (note the limited application to cerebrum, not the brain as a whole)
- supracostal (supra/cost/al)—situated above or upon a rib or ribs
- suprahepatic (supra/hepat/ic)—situated above the liver

There is a closely related prefix *super-* "the upper part of" or "excessive."

Examples:
- supercerebral (super/cerebr/al)—in the upper part of the cerebrum (compare supracerebral above)
- superacute (super/acute)—extremely acute
- superior (super/ior)—situated above; directed upward; in anatomy, used to designate the upper surface of an organ or other structure or to a structure occupying a higher position
- superofrontal (super/o/front/al)—situated at the upper and frontal part of a structure
- superolateral (super/o/later/al)—above and at the side (*later-* which is discussed in Lesson 9 means "side")
- superfunction (super/function)—excessive activity of an organ such as a gland; hyperfunctioning

trip- rub; friction *grinding*

> Examples:
> *crushing*
> • tripsis (trip/sis)—the act of rubbing, massaging

-tripsy (tripsy) is a word ending derived from the Greek element trip- that means crushing. It is used mainly to denote the medical procedure of crushing a calculous (stone):
> • lithotripsy (lith/o/trips/y)—crushing of a calculus (stone) within the bladder
> • hepaticolithotripsy (hepat/ic/o/lith/o/trips/y)—the operation of crushing a stone in a liver (hepat/ic) duct
> • cholecystolithotripsy (chole/cyst/o/lith/o/trips/y)—the crushing of gallstones (cholelith) in the gallbladder (cholecyst)

(e)

-trophy development, growth; nutrition, nourishment

> Examples:
> • trophic (troph/ic)—pertaining to nutrition, development, growth
> • trophopathy (troph/o/path/y)—any disease due to faulty nutrition
> • trophotherapy (troph/o/therap/y)—treatment of disease by nourishment (diet) measures

Some important combinations frequently appearing at the ends of medical words or phrases:
> • hypertrophy (hyper/trophy)—"over development"; the overgrowth of an organ or part
> • atrophy (a/trophy)—"not growth"; a wasting away or decrease in the size of cell, tissue, organ or body part (*a-* has a meaning "not," "without")
> • dystrophy (dys/trophy)—"bad development"; a disorder arising from defective or faulty nutrition (*dys-* means "bad" and is discussed more fully in Lesson 9)

Lesson 3—Element Recognition

Separate the word terminals, elements, and connecting vowels of the following medical terms from right to left by inserting a slash mark (/) between them.

Example: hydrocholecystitis—hydro/chole/cyst/itis

cost/o/chondral
cartilage in the ribs

chole/cyst/o/gram
record of the bladder bile

acro/path/o/logy
study of the disease of extremities

angi/o/rrhexis
rupture of vessels

carcin/o/gen/esis

hydropenia

path/o/gen

burso/lith

retrocervical

lithotripsy

arthrodesis

glossoplasty

autotrophy

supracerebral

blepharoptosis

myodynia

mastadenitis

glossorrhaphy

dentoid

cephalogenesis

autocystoplasty

epicystitis

hydrohepatosis

angiogram

acromegaly

cardiorrhexis

carcinoma

hypogenesis

bursopathy

retrocardiac

cephalopathy

autology

epidermis

hydrology

mania

glossalgia

trophology

supracostal

gastroptosis

cervicodynia

mastocarcinoma

myorrhaphy

Complete the following statements by printing the meanings of the elements that make up the medical term in the proper blanks. (Remember, most medical terms are interpreted from right to left.)

3-1.   Acrocyanosis (acro/cyan/osis) is a condition of _____ coloring of the _____.

3-2.   Autolysis (auto/lysis) refers to the _____ of tissue due to causes within the patients own _____.

3-3.   Bursitis (Burs/itis) is an _____ of the bursa that are closed _____ containing fluid that lay between surfaces that slide over one another.

3-4.   An adenocarcinoma (aden/o/carcin/oma) is a _____ _____ composed of _____-like cells.

3-5.   Cephalic (cephal/ic) is a term which means pertaining to , near or in the _____.

3-6.   The term chondrocostal (chondr/o/cost/al) denotes pertaining to or of the _____ and _____.

3-7.   The term dental (dent/al) means pertaining to or of the _____.

3-8.   Arthrodesis (arthr/o/desis) is the surgical _____ of a _____.

3-9.   The term epidermis (epi/derm/is) denotes pertaining to the _____ _____.

3-10.   A pathogen (path/o/gen) is a _____ of _____.

3-11.   Glossoscopy (glosso/scop/y) refers to the _____ of the _____.

3-12.   A cardiogram (cardi/o/gram) is a _____ of the _____.

3-13.   A hydrocyst (hydro/cyst) is a cyst or _____ filled with _____.

3-14.   The term megalomania (megal/o/mani/a) denotes an _____ with or for
_____.

3-15.   A mastectomy (mast/ectomy) is the surgical _____ of all or part of the
_____.

3-16.   The term acrodynia (acr/odyn/ia) denotes _____ in the _____.

3-17.   Hydropenia (hydro/penia) denotes a _____ of _____ in the body.

3-18.   Blepharoptosis (blephar/o/ptosis) refers to the _____ of an _____.

3-19.   The term retrocardiac (retro/cardi/ac) denotes pertaining to _____the
_____.

3-20.   The term myorrhaphy (my/o/rrhaphy) denotes a _____ of a _____.

3-21   The term hysterorrhexis (hyster/o/rrhexis) denotes a _____of the
_____.

3-22.   Streptococcus (strept/o/coccus) is the name of an infectious microorganism so called
because of its _____ form.

3-23.   Suprahepatic (supra/hepat/ic) means pertaining to or of a location _____
the _____.

3-24.   The term lithotripsy (lith/o/trips/y) denotes the _____of a _____
most often in the urinary bladder.

3-25   Hypertrophy (hyper/trophy) denotes _____ _____.

Lesson 4

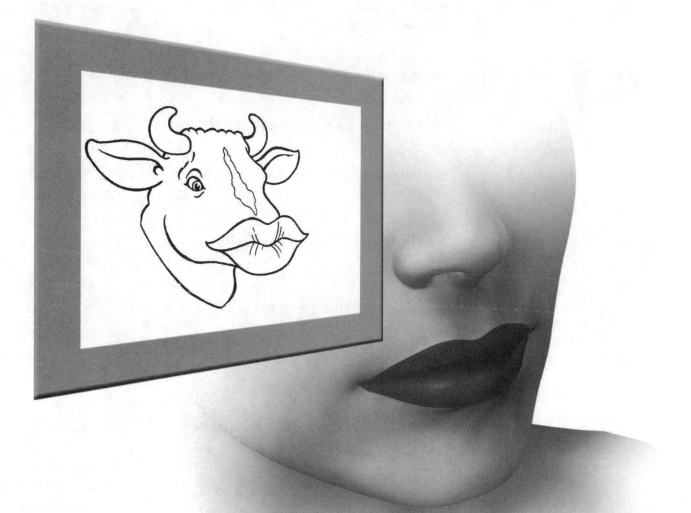

Lesson 4—Review

Element	Audionym	Visual Image	Meaning
lobo-	low bow	See the **low bow** made of **section**s!	section
-emesis	Hey Mrs.	See the bellhop saying, **"Hey Mrs.!"** as she is **vomiting** in the lobby!	vomiting
contra-	contractor	See the **contra**ctor leaning the tools **against** the **counter**!	against, counter
-iasis	oasis	See the **oasis** with air-**conditioner**s on it!	condition
trans-	trains	See the **trains** going **through a cross**!	through, across
brady-	braid	See the girl's hair being **braid**ed so **slow**ly she grows old!	slow
-ectasis	egged a sis	See the boy who **"egged a sis"** with an **"X" pan**!	expansion
cyt-	sight	See the **sight** of the gun made of a **cell**!	cell
odont-	Oh don't	See the person saying "**Oh don't** hit me with that **tooth**"!	tooth
leuk-	Look (Look Magazine)	See the **Look** Magazine that is all **white**!	white
-esthesia	has the show	See the man who h**as the sh**ow (holding the stage). He is **sensation**al!	sensation
cantho-	can throw	See the **can** being **thrown** at the **angle at the end of the eyelid**!	angle at the end of the eyelid

Element	Audionym	Visual Image	Meaning
steno-	stenographer	See the **steno**grapher typing a **narrow contract**!	narrow, contracted
cheil-	cow	See the **cow** with human **lip**s!	lip
-cele	seal	See the **seal** on **her knee**!	hernia
benign	bee 9	See the **bee** stinging the **"9"** that **mel**ts into a k**not** and falls into a **can**!	mild, not cancerous
semen	seaman	See the **seaman** with his hat filled with **seed**s!	seed
celio-	ceiling dome	See the **ceili**ng dome with an ap**ple dome** hanging from it!	abdomen
erythro-	wreath throw	See the **wreath** being **throw**n change to **red**!	red
vaso-	vase	See the **vase** with **vessel**s all over it!	vessel
melan-	melon	See the **melon** that is **black**!	black
cauda-	cod liver oil	See the **cod** liv**er** oil with a **tail** sticking out of it!	tail
lingua-	language	See the man who speaks many **language**s because he has many **tongue**s!	tongue
myring-	my ring	See **"my ring"** with an **ear** and a **drum** on it!	eardrum
spondyl-	spun doll	See the **spun doll** spinning so fast that you can see the **spinal column**!	spinal column

Lesson 4—Worksheet

Print the audionym and meaning of the elements in the proper blanks:

Element	Audionym	Meaning
lobo-	low bow	section
-emesis *	Hey Mrs	vomiting
contra-	contractor	against, counter
-iasis	oasis	condition
trans-	train	through, across
brady-	braid	slow
-ectasis	egged a sis	expansion
cyt-	sight	cell
odont-	o don't	tooth
leuk-	look magazine	white
-esthesia	has the show	sensation
cantho-	can thro	media corner of the eye
steno-		
cheil-		
-cele *		
benign *		
semen *		
celio- *		
erythro-		
vaso-		
melan-		
cauda-		
lingua-		
myring-		
spondyl-		

Lesson 4—Word Terminals

-a	noun ending; used to form the name of a thing from a root

Examples:
- derma (derm/a)— the skin
- gingiva (gingiv/a)—the gum
- costa (cost/a)—a rib

Also, the terminal to form the plural of words ending in *-on* and *-um.*

Examples:
- bacteri/um—bacteri/a; dat/um—dat/a; criteri/on—criteri/a; phenomen/on—phenomen/a

-ae	plural ending for words ending in *-a*

Examples:
- gingiv/a—gingiv/ae; cost/a—cost/ae; burs/a— burs/ae

-ant	pertaining to; having the characteristics of

Examples:
- pleasant (pleas/ant)—having the characteristics of pleasing
- malignant (malign/ant)—having the characteristics of badness

-ation	a process, action, or condition

This terminal is a combination of *-ate* (to put into action) and *-ion* (condition resulting from an action).

Examples:
- starv/ation, observ/ation, discolor/ation, decor/ation

-esis	condition or process

Examples:
- genesis (gen/esis)—the process of producing or originating
- uresis (ur/esis)—the process of passing urine (the element *ur-* means "urine")

☞ **Note:** The terminal *-esis* is closely related to the element *-osis* (Lesson 1).

| *-ics* | the body of facts, knowledge, matters, etc., pertaining to a subject and hence a science or art; the study of |

Examples:
- polit/ics, mathemat/ics, electron/ics, opt/ics, athlet/ics, econom/ics

☞ **Note:** *-ics* carries a meaning identical with *-ology*. However, there is a subtle distinction in medicine. When *-ics* and *-ology* are used to denote a body of medical knowledge, the *-ology* ending is used for the field covered by the doctor of medicine or osteopathy; the *-ics* is limited to the non-M.D. or D.O. field.

Anesthesiology is the broad field covered by the medical doctor (M.D.); anesthetics is the field covered by the non-M.D., usually a technician.

Ophthalmology is the field covered by the M.D.; optics is the field covered by the non-M.D.

| *-in* | organic compounds such as carbohydrates and protein |

Example:
- melanin (melan/in)—an organic compound providing a dark color to skin and hair

| *-ly* | in a manner, in a way, by way of, toward |

Examples:
- slowly (slow/ly)—in a slow manner
- smilingly (smiling/ly)—in a smiling way
- lingually (lingual/ly)—toward the tongue, by way of the tongue

| *-tic* | pertaining to |

This terminal is especially used to give a "pertaining to" meaning to words ending in *-sis*.

Examples:
- eme/sis—eme/tic; analy/sis—analy/tic; diagno/sis—diagnos/tic; hypno/sis—hypno/tic

Lesson 4—Reading Assignment

---

benign   mild; not cancerous / not recurrent; favorable for recovery

This word is used in phrases to describe the relative severity of a disease.

Examples:
- mild vs. severe as in "a benign psychosis"
- not threatening life or health as in "a benign malaria"
- having a good prognosis (a forecast as to the probable result of an attack of disease; the prospect as to recovery from a disease) as in "a benign psychosis"

The principal use of the word is to designate the absence of cancerous tumors as in "a benign tumor" versus "a carcin/oma."

---

brady-   slow / slowness; abnormal slowness in physical or mental process

This root is descriptive and can practically always be interpreted as "slowness of" or "abnormal slowness of."

Examples:
- bradycardia (brady/card/ia)—abnormal slowness of the heartbeat (usually less than 60 beats per minute)
- myobradia (my/o/brad/ia)—a slow, sluggish reaction of muscle to electrical stimulation

An interesting illustration of the use of roots to describe different causes for similar symptoms is the symptom "abnormal slowness of speech":
- bradyglossia (brady/glossia)—abnormal slowness of utterance (the vocal forming of sounds to express speech)
- bradylogia (brady/log/ia)—abnormal slowness of speech due to slowness of thinking as in a mental disorder

☞ **Note:** Difficulty in physically forming words is conveyed by the use of *gloss-* (tongue), the principal organ used in the forming of speech sounds. On the other hand, the use of *log-* (*-ology*, "study of") carries the idea of a mental process. (The application of the element *log-* for the mental process makes more sense when we know that the original meaning of *log-* was "discourse" or "speaking on." An *-ologist*, a "student of" a subject, had the ability to "speak on" the subject.)

cantho-   angle at the end of the eyelid; one of the corners of the eye; either of the angles formed by the meeting of the upper and lower eyelids

Examples:
- canthal (canth/al)—pertaining to a corner of the eye
- canthus (canth/us)—name of the corner of the eye

The tissue forming the corner of the eye may become inflamed, incised, excised, repaired, or loosened. Can you form the appropriate medical terms for these conditions and procedures?

cauda-   tail / tail part of the body; the "rear end"; a tail-like appendage (something hanging upon a main structure; the "appendix" is a small pouch or sac "hanging on" to a section of the intestines)

Examples:
- caudal (caud/al)—pertaining to the tail (the "rear end") or a tail-like appendage; pertaining to the lower and/or rear end
- cauda (caud/a)—name for a tail-like appendage

This root is used principally to indicate a direction, a position toward the tail ("rear end") of the body or a body part. It may also be used to name a tail-like appendage.

Examples:
- caudad (caud/ad)—directed toward a cauda or tail; opposite to cephal/ad
- caudalward (caud/al/ward)—toward the caudal, tail or back end
- caudal anesthesia (caud/al an/esthesia)—loss of sensation produced by an injection of an anesthetic into the lower (caudal) portion of the spinal cord

-cele   hernia, tumor or swelling / an external projection of a part from its natural cavity

In Lesson 3, we learned that the suffix *-rhexis* named a condition of breaking, bursting, rupturing. The physical evidence of such a rupturing or breaking out is a hernia, frequently a balloon-like protrusion of an organ through its containing wall. *-Cele* is the suffix used to denote a hernia.

Examples:
- myocele (my/o/cele)—a muscle hernia; a muscle protrusion
- cystocele (cyst/o/cele)—protrusion of the bladder through the vaginal wall
- cephalocele (cephal/o/cele)—protrusion of part of the cranial contents
- hydrocele (hydr/o/cele)—collection of fluid in a swelling; especially in male genital parts

celio- abdomen; any large cavity of the body, especially the abdomen

Examples:

- celiac (celi/ac)—pertaining to the abdomen
- celiorrhaphy (celio/rrhaphy)—suture of the abdominal wall
- celitis (cel/itis)—any inflammation of the abdomen
- celiotomy (celi/otomy)—surgical incision into the abdominal cavity

cheil- lip / the lips of the face; infrequently used to denote an edge or brim

Examples:

- cheilocarcinoma (cheil/o/carcin/oma)—cancer of the lip
- cheilorrhaphy (cheil/o/rrhaphy)—suturing of the lips
- cheiloplasty (cheil/o/plast/y)—surgical repair of the lips
- cheilosis (cheil/osis)—a condition of the lips characterized by chapping and fissuring

contra- against; counter / in opposition to; a thing opposite or against another

This prefix may be attached to a word or stem with the meaning "opposite to" or "against."

Examples:

- contraction (contr/action)—"acting against"; a shortening; for example, a muscle contraction
- contraception (contra/ception)—"acting against conception"; the prevention of pregnancy
- contrastimulant (contra/stimulant)—"against stimulation"; a medicine or action applied to overcome or alleviate stimulation

Counter- which has the same meaning of "against" or "opposite to" is used frequently to indicate "a direction opposite to."

Examples:

- counteropening (counter/opening) (also counter/incision)—a second incision made opposite to another, as in an abscess, to promote drainage
- counterirritation (counter/irritation)—an irritation which is supposed to relieve some other irritation

cyt- cell / a small, usually microscopic mass of sticky fluid contained in a membranous sac

This root is widely used in medicine since it means "cell." Cells are the building blocks of the body. All body parts consist of tissues that are made up of cells. Cells of one tissue differ from those of other tissues depending on the function they perform.

Examples:

- hemocyte or hemacyte (hem/o/cyt/e, hema/cyt/e)—a blood cell; blood cells are of two kinds:
  - leukocyte (leuk/o/cyt/e)—white blood cell
  - erythrocyte (erythr/o/cyt/e)—red blood cell
- myocyte (my/o/cyt/e)—a cell of the muscular tissue
- -cytic (-cyt/ic)—pertaining to cells
- cytogenesis (cyt/o/gen/esis)—the production and development of cells

-ectasis   expansion / "a stretching out"; enlargement

This suffix denotes an enlargement (in a limited sense, a *-megaly*) by stretching; the condition of being stretched beyond normal dimensions (*ec-* a variation of *ex-* meaning "out" + tasis "stretching").

Examples:

- angiectasis (angi/ectasis)—beyond normal stretching of a blood vessel
- nephrectasis (nephr/ectasis)—stretching (distention) of the kidney

Another way of expressing "ectasis" is the word "dilatation." You probably know that dilate means "to expand," "to stretch." In medical terms dilatation means "the condition of being dilated or stretched beyond normal dimensions."

-emesis   vomiting / a condition or occurrence ("happening") of vomiting

Our clue here is the ending *-sis* meaning "condition." Therefore, this must mean a condition of "eme-." Since we learned that *-emesis* means "vomiting," the "eme" must mean "vomit" and so it does. *Eme-* is a root meaning "vomit." *-Emesis* is used as a suffix combination or as a word.

Examples:

- emesis (eme/sis)— the act of vomiting
- emetic (eme/tic)—that which causes vomiting such as a drug
- emeticology (eme/tic/ology)—also emetology (emet/ology)— the study of, or that which causes vomiting
- hematemesis (hemat/eme/sis)—the vomiting of blood
- cholemesis (chol/eme/sis)—the vomiting of bile or gall

erythro-   red / the color red

Examples:

- erythra (erythr/a)—an eruption (breaking out) of the skin marked by redness of the skin and/or swelling
- erythralgia (erythr/algia)—a condition marked by pain and redness of the skin
- erythrocyt- (erythr/o/cyt-)—meaning "red cell," actually "red blood cell," is a

frequent combination in medical terms:

- erythrocytopenia (erythr/o/cyt/o/penia)—deficiency of the number of red blood cells; frequently shortened to erythropenia
- erythrocythemia (erythr/o/cyt/hem/ia)—a condition of increase of the number of red blood cells; also erythrocytosis

-esthesia   sensation, feeling / perception; physical sensitivity; consciousness

Examples:

- -esthetic (-esthet/ic)—pertaining to feeling
- -esthesia (-esthes/ia)—the condition of feeling; a "feeling of"; awareness of feeling
- optesthesia (opt/esthesia)—the ability to see; the ability to perceive visual stimuli

This root, in medical terms, deals primarily with physical sensations, particularly the sense of pain and the general feeling of the senses (consciousness, perception). An important derivative of *esthes-* is its opposite *an/esthes-* "lack of feeling" or absence of feeling (*an-* "lack of" covered in Lesson 10).

Examples:

- anesthesia (an/esthesia)—the condition of lack of feeling
- anesthesiology (an/esthesi/ology)—the branch of medical science dealing with the bringing about the loss of sensation, principally as an adjunct to pain-causing therapeutic procedures such as surgery

-iasis   condition; formation of; presence of / state of (almost always relating to disease or abnormality)

This suffix is widely used in medicine to denote a disease process or the condition resulting from disease, literally "illness condition" or "sick condition." In Lesson 1 you learned that the word ending *-ia* means disease.

Examples:

- lithiasis (lith/iasis)—a condition characterized by the formation of stones
- elephantiasis (elephant/iasis)—a condition characterized by enlargement of the parts affected and thickening and discoloration of the skin covering these parts

leuk-   white / the color white

Examples:

- leukemia, leukocythemia (leuk/em/ia, leuk/o/cyt/hem/ia)—a frequently fatal condition in which there is an overproduction of white blood cells in the tissues (hem, em = blood)
- leukocyte (leuk/o/cyt/e)—a white (colorless) blood cell
- leukocyt- (leuk/o/cyt-)—combining form meaning white blood cell

Because there are so many morbid conditions characterized by an increase in the number of leukocytes in the blood, a variety of suffixes may be attached to this stem:

- leukocytosis (leuk/o/cyt/osis)—a condition of increased leukocytes in the blood
- leukocytoma (leuk/o/cyt/oma)—a tumorlike mass of leukocytes

---

lingua   tongue / the tongue; name for the tongue of the mouth

Examples:
- lingual (lingu/al)—pertaining to the tongue
- lingula (ling/ula)—a small tongue; generally a part of the body which is shaped like and projects like a tongue
- lingually (lingu/al/ly)—toward the tongue

This root means the same as *gloss-* (Lesson 3) in that both refer to the tongue in the mouth. However, they are used for different purposes. *Lingu-* is mostly used to designate the tongue as a structure, a point of reference (landmark):

- retrolingual (retr/o/lingu/al)—behind the tongue

Gloss- is the root which is principally used to denote diseases, injuries and the therapeutic procedures used for the alleviation of such diseases and injuries.

---

lobo-   section / a more or less well-defined portion of any organ, especially of the brain and glands

Examples:
- lobe (lob/e)—name for a well-defined portion of an organ; organs having such parts are the brain, the lungs, the liver, the glands, the ears
- lobule (lob/ule)—a small lobe
- lobectomy (lob/ectomy)—excision of a lobe, as of the thyroid, liver, brain or lung
- lobar (lob/ar)—of or pertaining to a lobe or section

---

melan-   black / the color black

Examples:
- melanin (melan/in)—a black or dark brown pigment in the skin and hair
- melanocyte (melan/o/cyt/e)—the cell responsible for the production of black pigment
- melanodermic, melanous (melan/o/derm/ic, melan/ous)—having a dark skin
- melanemia (melan/em/ia)—a condition in which the blood contains a black or dark brown pigment
- melanosis (melan/osis)—a condition characterized by abnormal deposits of black pigment; also called melan/ism
- cardiomelanosis (cardi/o/melan/osis)—deposits of black pigment in the heart; melanosis of the heart

myring- eardrum / the sheet of membrane forming a partition between the outer and inner ear

Examples:
- myringa (myring/a)—the eardrum; name of the eardrum
- myringoscopy (myring/o/scop/y)—inspection of the eardrum using a myringoscope
- myringoplasty (myring/o/plast/y)—surgical repair of defects of the eardrum

odont- tooth

Examples:
- odontic, odontal (odont/ic, odont/al)—pertaining to a tooth/pertaining to the teeth
- -odontia (-odont/ia)—form, condition or mode of treatment of the teeth
- odontogenic (odont/o/gen/ic)—originating in the teeth
- endodontics (end/odont/ics)—the branch of dentistry dealing with the inside of the tooth including the cause, prevention, diagnosis and treatment of diseases affecting the inner structure of a tooth, principally the pulp which fills the inside of the root canals; also called endodontia

semen seed / the name of the thick, whitish secretion of the male reproductive organs that carries and transfers the sperm for fertilization of the egg in the female reproductive system

Example:
- semenology (semen/ology)—the study of semen

The root may also appear in the form *semin-:*
- seminal (semin/al)—pertaining to the semen
- semination (semin/ation)—production or dispersal of semen; seed

The term semination is used more definitively with the prefix - *in*, (in/semin/ation), to indicate dispersal or introduction of semen into the uterus or genital tract of a female as in intercourse.

spondyl- spinal column or vertebra; vertebra, a bone of the spine; spinal column, the "back bone"

This root is used to denote the spinal column, that is the structure consisting of a series of twenty-six jointed bones (vertebrae) beginning at the back of the head, extending through the neck and back, and ending at the tailbone (the last vertebrae.) It is also used to denote any one of the twenty-six bones (a vertebra; plural, the vertebrae) of the back.

Examples:
- spondylic, spondylous (spondyl/ic, spondyl/ous)—pertaining to a vertebra; pertaining to the spinal column

Spondyl-, in common with many of the other body parts that you have learned, can carry a variety of suffixes to denote morbid conditions or therapeutic procedures. Can you form the words which would mean "pain in," "inflammation of," "incision into," "any disease of," "puncture of?"

It's obvious that the column formed by these twenty-six bones must be jointed. Can you form the combination which would carry the meaning "inflammation of spinal joint(s)?"

steno-	narrow; contracted / constricted; close

This descriptive root can apply to a body structure to express less than normal width:

- stenocephalous (steno/cephal/ous)—having a narrow head
- stenocephalia (steno/cephal/ia)—excessive narrowness of the head
- stenostomia (steno/stom/ia)—narrowing of the mouth

Stenosis (steno/sis) is a word meaning constriction of a passage in the body such as a duct or canal thus producing a narrowing that interferes with passage of material through the tubelike passage:

- stenosis or -stenosis (steno/sis, -steno/sis)—narrowing of a duct or canal
- angiostenosis (angi/o/steno/sis)—narrowing of the diameter of a vessel
- enterostenosis (enter/o/steno/sis)—narrowing of the intestine

Stricture is a word that is also applied in medicine to denote abnormal narrowing of a canal, duct or passage either from the build up of healing tissue, such as scar tissue, the deposit of normal tissue, inflammation (swelling) or as the result of a spasm.

trans-	through; across; beyond / to the other side

The "through" idea of the prefix *trans-* is encountered frequently in the description of operating techniques to describe the approach being made:

- transdermic (trans/derm/ic)— through the skin

The "across" idea is illustrated in actions involving a "movement across," a "carrying across," a "transfer":

- transfusion (trans/fus/ion)—(*fus-* means "to pour") the introduction of blood from another source; a "pouring across" of blood
- transplant (trans/plant)—a piece of tissue for grafting taken from another part of the patient's body or from a donor; a "planting across"

The "beyond" application, frequently carrying the idea of "more than," is seen in:

- transnormal (trans/normal)—beyond normal, more than normal

> ***vaso-***   vessel / any canal for carrying fluid; a duct; a channel; but, principally a blood vessel or lymph vessel

Here is another case in which we have two roots that are synonyms, *vas-* and *angi-* (Lesson 1) both of which mean vessel, especially a blood vessel. Although there is overlapping in their applications to medical terminology, for the most part, *vas-* is used in naming the various ailments affecting vessels and the therapy taken to overcome or correct such ailments.

Examples:

- vascular (vas/cul/ar)—pertaining to a vessel; full of vessels
- vasculum (vas/cul/um)—a small vessel
- cerebrovascular (cerebr/o/vas/cul/ar)—pertaining to the blood vessels of the cerebrum or brain
- myovascular (my/o/vas/cul/ar)—pertaining to the muscle and its blood vessels
- vasectomy (vas/ectomy)—surgical excision of all or part of the duct in the male through which the sperm is secreted

Lesson 4—Element Recognition

Separate the word terminals, elements, and connecting vowels of the following medical terms from right to left by inserting a slash mark (/) between them.

Example: gastrolithiasis—gastr/o/lith/iasis

lobotomy	lingual
emetology	spondylodynia
contraception	leukoderma
odontiasis	canthorrhaphy
transdermic	cheilitis
bradyglossia	cystocele
angiectasis	celioma
cytopathology	erythropenia
odontotripsis	vasalgia
leukocytopenia	melanoderma
hyperesthesia	myringoplasty
cantholysis	spondylolysis
stenocephaly	lobectomy
cheiloplasty	lithiasis
enterocele	transfusion
semenologist	bradycardia
celialgia	cardiectasis
erythrocyanosis	cytogenesis
vasorrhaphy	odontoptosis
melanocarcinoma	cheilotomy
caudal	myringoscope

Lesson 4—Interpretation Exercise

Complete the following statements by printing the meanings of the elements that make up the medical term in the proper blanks. (Remember, most medical terms are interpreted from right to left.)

4-1.   A benign tumor is a _____ tumor.

4-2.   Bradycardia (brady/card/ia) denotes an abnormally _____ _____.

4-3.   The term canthal (canth/al) denotes pertaining to the _____ of the eye.

4-4.   The term caudalward (caud/al/ward) indicates towards the _____ end.

4-5.   A myocele (my/o/cele) is a _____ _____.

4-6.   A celiotomy (celi/otomy) is the surgical procedure of making an _____ into the _____ cavity.

4-7.   A cheilocarcinoma (cheil/o/carcin/oma) is a _____ _____ of the _____.

4-8.   The term contrastimulant (contra/stimulant) means _____ stimulation.

4-9.   A hemocyte (hem/o/cyt/e) is a _____ _____.

4-10.   The term angiectasis (angi/ectasis) denotes the beyond normal _____ of a _____.

4-11.   The term cholemesis (chol/emesis) denotes the _____ of _____.

4-12.   Erythrocytopenia (erythr/o/cyt/o/penia) denotes a _____ of _____ blood _____.

4-13.   Anesthesiology (an/esthesi/ology) is the branch of medicine that specializes in the

_____ of bringing about the loss of _____.

4-14.   Lithiasis (lith/iasis) is a _____ characterized by the formation

of _____.

4-15.   A leukocyte (leuk/o/cyt/e) is a _____ blood _____.

4-16.   The term lingual (lingu/al) denotes pertaining to or of the _____.

4-17.   A lobotomy (lob/otomy) is a surgical _____ of a _____.

4-18.   Melanosis (melan/osis) is a _____ characterized by abnormal deposits of

_____ pigment.

4-19.   Myringoscopy (myring/o/scop/y/) is the _____ of the _____

using a myringoscope.

4-20.   The term odontic (odont/ic) pertains to or of the _____.

4-21.   Semenology (semen/ology) is the _____ of _____.

4-22.   The term spondylous (spondyl/ous) means pertaining to or of a _____ or the

_____.

4-23.   Stenosis (steno/sis) is a term that denotes a _____ of _____

usually of a duct or canal.

4-24.   The term transdermic (trans/derm/ic) pertains to _____ the _____.

4-25.   A vasodilator (vaso/dilator) causes the _____ of a blood _____.

Lesson 5

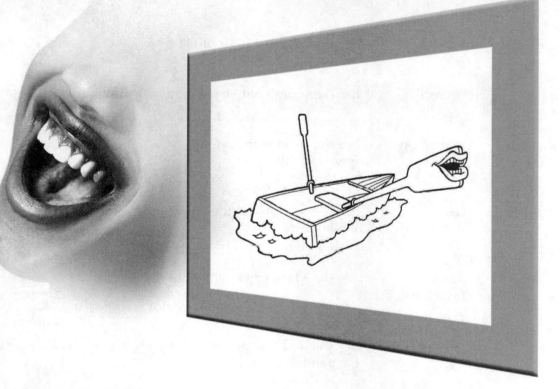

Lesson 5—Review

Element	Audionym	Visual Image	Meaning
ovar-	over	See the **over**turned **egg** and an **egg** being turned **over**!	egg (egg, the female reproductive cell)
-centesis	cent	See the **cent** being **punctured**!	puncture
oto-	"O" toe	See the **"O" to**e with an **ear** growing out of it!	ear
bili-	bill	See the **bill**s in a high **pile**!	bile
squam-	squash	See the **squa**sh with a **scale** bursting out of it!	scale
mening-	managing	See the woman **manag**ing **men's brain**s!	membrane
cec-	seek	See the person **seek**ing a **passage** while **blind**folded!	blind passage
macul-	Mack (Mack truck)	See the **Mack** truck with **spot**s all over it!	spot
-pexy	pecks egg	See the bird that **pecks** the **egg** while **suspended** in the air!	suspension
onco-	uncle	See the image of **uncle** and see **tw**o **more**!	tumor
or-	oar	See the **oar** with a **mouth** on it!	mouth
sub-	submarine	See the **sub**marine sandwich **under** the water!	under
spiro-	sparrow	See the **sparro**w made of **coil**s!	coil

Lesson 5

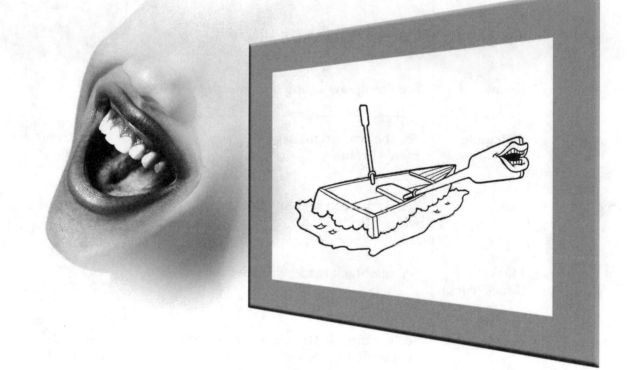

Lesson 5—Review

Element	Audionym	Visual Image	Meaning
ovar-	over	See the **over**turned **egg** and an **egg** being turned **over**!	egg (egg, the female reproductive cell)
-centesis	cent	See the **cent** being **punctured**!	puncture
oto-	"O" toe	See the **"O" toe** with an **ear** growing out of it!	ear
bili-	bill	See the **bill**s in a high **pile**!	bile
squam-	squaw	See the **squaw** sitting on the **scale**!	scale
mening-	managing	See the woman **manag**ing **men**'s **brain**s!	membrane
cec-	seek	See the person **seek**ing a **passage** while **blind**folded!	blind passage
macul-	Mack (Mack truck)	See the **Mack** truck with **spot**s all over it!	spot
-pexy	pecks egg	See the bird that **pecks** the **egg** while **suspended** in the air!	suspension
onco-	uncle	See the image of **uncle** and see **two more**!	tumor
or-	oar	See the **oar** with a **mouth** on it!	mouth
sub-	submarine	See the **sub**marine sandwich **under** the water!	under
spiro-	sparrow	See the **sparro**w made of **coil**s!	coil

Lesson 5—Review

Element	Audionym	Visual Image	Meaning
lacrim-	lake rim	See the **lake rim** with a gigantic **tear** on it!	**tear**
viscero-	vice row	See the person on the **vice ro**wing with **organ**s!	organ
lact-	lacquer	See the image of **lac**quer and see **milk** being used instead!	milk
onych-	onyx	See the **onyx** ring with a **nail** and a **claw** stuck in it!	nail, claw
thorac-	throw rack	See the person **thro**wing a **rac**k with a treasure **chest** hanging on it!	chest
pyle-	pie	See the **pie** with a **gate** on it!	gate
vesic-	vest sick	See the **ves**t that is **sic**k. It is made of a **bladder**!	bladder
sphenic-	sphinx	See the **sphin**x shaped like a **wedge**!	wedge
myel-	mile (mile sign)	See the **mile** sign supported by a **narrow spinal cord**!	marrow, spinal cord
anti-	ant eye	See the **ant**'s **eye against** the rock!	against
myco-	my comb	See "**my co**mb" covered with **fungus**!	fungus
hallux	hall "X"	See the **hall** shaped like an **"X"** with a **great toe** at the ends of each hall!	great toe (big toe)

Print the audionym and meaning of the elements in the proper blanks:

Element	Audionym	Meaning
ovar-	over - egg	egg container
-centesis	cent	puncture
oto-	O toe	ear
bili-	billy - pile	bile
squam-	squaw	scale
mening-		membrain
cec-	seek	
macul-	mack truck	spot
-pexy	pecks egg - suspended	suspension
onco-	uncle - two more	tumor
or-	oar	mouth
sub-	submarine	under
spiro-	sparrow	coil
lacrim-	lake rim	tear
viscero	vise row	organ
lact-	lacture	milk
onych-	onyx	nail / claw
thorac-	throw rack	chest
pyle-, pyloro-		gate
vesic-	vest sick	bladder
sphenic-	sphenx	wedge
myel-	mile	marrow, spinal cord
anti-	ant eye	against
myco-	my comb	fungus
hallux-	nail x	big toe

Lesson 5—Word Terminals

| **-es** | plural ending similar to -s |

Examples:
- kiss—kisses; fish—fishes; meninx (membrane)—meninges (membranes)

| **-id** | pertaining to; "being" |

Examples:
- fluid (flu/id)—to flow
- frigid (frig/id)—to be cold
- rigid (rig/id)—to be stiff
- parotid (par/ot/id)—being near the ear

| **-ness** | state; quality; instance of being |

Examples:
- great/ness, sad/ness, together/ness, loneli/ness, good/ness, sick/ness

| **-us** | noun ending; used to form the name of a thing from the root |

Example:
- disc/us

Lesson 5—Reading Assignment

anti- against / opposing; counteracting (acting against); inhibiting; preventing; suppressing; neutralizing or destroying; relieving

This prefix is widely used in medical terms as it is in common words with the broad meaning "against."

Examples:
- antigen (anti/gen)—a substance that, when introduced into the body, stimulates the "production of" an "opposing" substance called an anti/body
- antibody (anti/body)—a physical substance either in the body or produced by the action of an antigen which will prevent, relieve, or destroy the effect of infections or poisonous substances in the blood or tissues
- antacid (ant/acid)—a substance that counteracts or neutralizes acidity
- antiemetic (anti/emet/ic)—preventing or relieving nausea and vomiting
- anticoagulant (anti/coagulant)—a substance that suppresses or opposes the coagulation of the blood

bili- bile / gall; a thick, sticky yellow or greenish fluid secreted by the liver and flowing into the intestines where it is mixed with gastric fluids to aid digestion, particularly in the breaking down of fats; *chole-*

Gallbladder, bile cyst, cholecyst—names for the sac or pouch in which bile is stored.

Examples:
- biliary (bili/ary)—pertaining to the bile or pertaining collectively to the bile, bile ducts, and gallbladder:
  - biliary canal (bili/ary)—a tube (duct) through which the bile passes from the liver; hepatic duct; biliary duct
  - biliary tract (bili/ary)—the region that secretes and transmits bile; the bile duct and gallbladder
- biliousness (bili/ous/ness)—a discomfort characterized by constipation, headache, and indigestion, attributed to an excess production of bile

cec- a blind passage

A blind passage, like a "blind alley" is a space having only one outlet so that passage or flow cannot occur all the way through. Although the root may be used to refer to any such passage in the body, it is applied most frequently to denote the cecum.

The cecum (cec/um) is a large pouch at the beginning of the large intestine with only one opening. Incidentally, the appendix hangs at the end of the cecum.

As is true with other pouches in the body, the cecum may be:

- cut—cecotomy (cec/otomy)
- partially "cut out"—cecectomy (cec/ectomy)
- provided with a mouth or artificial opening—cecostomy (cec/ostomy)
- sutured—cecorrhaphy (cec/o/rrhaphy)
- fixed (usually to the abdominal wall)—cecopexy (cec/o/pexy)

The operations performed may be the result of conditions of disease or injury affecting the cecum:

- cecoptosis (cec/o/ptosis)—falling (downward displacement)
- cecitis (cec/itis)—inflammation
- cecorrhexis (cec/o/rrhexis)—rupturing; the cecorrhexis may have produced a hernia (cec/o/cele)
- cecal (cec/al)—pertaining to the cecum

-centesis   puncture / surgical puncture or incision, usually for the purpose of drainage

Examples:
- arthrocentesis (arthr/o/centesis)—surgical puncture of a joint
- cardicentesis (cardi/centesis)—surgical puncture or incision of the heart
- pericardicentesis (peri/cardi/centesis)—surgical puncture of the tissues surrounding the heart (the peri/cardi/um)

hallux   great toe / big toe

This is the medical name for the big toe or the great toe; also called the first digit of the foot. The fingers and toes are called digits and are numbered from the great toe in the case of the foot and the thumb in the case of the hand. Thus, hallux = great toe = big toe = first digit of the foot that may be the first digit of the right foot (big toe of the right foot) or the first digit of the left foot (big toe of the left foot).

lacrim-   tear / the tears; tears of the eye

Examples:
- lacrimal (sometimes lachrymal) (lacrim/al, lachrym/al)—pertaining to tears; relating to or situated near the organs that produce tears
- lacrimal glands (lacrim/al)—the glands that secrete tears
- lacrimal ducts (lacrim/al)—a term for ducts (canals, tubes) conveying the secretion (tears) of the lacrimal glands to the corner of the eye (canthus)
- lacrimotomy (lacrim/otomy)—incision of the lacrimal duct

lact-   milk / the fluid secretion of the gland of the breast in the female forming the natural food of infants

Examples:
- lacteal (lact/e/al)—pertaining to milk
- lactation (lact/ation)—the secretion of milk; suckling by infants
- lactogenic (lact/o/gen/ic)—stimulating the production of milk

- lactigenous (lact/i/gen/ous)— producing or secreting milk
- superlactation (super/lact/ation)—secretion of milk in greater than normal amount or for a longer than usual period

---

macul-   spot (or stain) / blotch; spotty or blotchy discoloration, especially of the skin

Examples:
- macula (macul/a)—a spot or blotch
- macule (macul/e)—a macula
- maculation (macul/ation)—the condition of being spotted; the formation of spots or macules

☞   **Note:** Tumors (*-oma, onc-*) are usually discolored but are always characterized by swelling. A macule is a discolored spot or patch that is flat, that is neither swollen or depressed. Birthmarks and freckles are examples of macules that are usually not a sign of disease. Macula, that are indicative of disease, are the spots that appear in some of the infectious diseases such as smallpox and leprosy; psoriasis and some poisons also produce spotty discolorations.

---

mening-   membrane / the membranes covering the brain and the spinal cord (myel-)

Examples:
- meningeal (mening/e/al)—pertaining to the meninges
- meninges (mening/es)—name for the membranous sheath that envelops the brain and spinal cord
- meningoencephal- (mening/o/encephal-)—form for the meninges and the brain or the meninges and brainy substance
- meningitis (mening/itis)—inflammation of the membranes covering the brain and spinal cord (the meninges)
  - cerebral meningitis (cerebr/al mening/itis)—inflammation of the meninges of the brain

---

myco-   fungus / relating to an infection with a fungus (a kind of plant that can form a destructive pathogen [disease producer] in humans and other animals)

Examples:
- mycete (myc/ete)—a fungus
- mycosis, -mycosis (myc/osis)—"a condition of fungus (infection)"; any disease caused by a fungus
- mycetoma, -mycetoma (myc/et/oma, -myc/et/oma)—a tumor containing fungus cells (mycetocytes)
- dermatomycosis (dermat/o/myc/osis)—a fungus infection of the skin that includes the conditions commonly called "athlete's foot" and "ring worm"
- acromycosis (acr/o/myc/osis)—a condition of fungus infection of the extremities (limbs)

myel- marrow (spinal cord) / the soft inner part of a bone; the cablelike tissue enclosed in the canal or tube formed by the bones of the spine (the vertebrae)

Examples:

- meningomyel- (mening/o/myel-)—form for the spinal cord and its membranous covering; also myel/o/mening/o-
- osteomyel- (oste/o/myel-)—form for bone marrow or the bone and its marrow
- osteomyelitis (oste/o/myel/itis)—inflammation of the bone and the bone marrow
- encephalomyel- (en/cephal/o/myel-)—form for the brain and the spinal cord; also myel/o/en/cephal
- encephalomyelopathy (en/cephal/o/myel/o/path/y)—any disease or diseased condition of the brain and spinal cord
- myeloencephalitis (myel/o/en/cephal/itis)—inflammation of the brain and spinal cord

☞ **Note:** The marrow of the bone and the spinal cord have structural similarities in that they are both surrounded by bone: bone marrow being the soft tissue filling the hollow interior of a bone; the spinal cord being a covered (mening-) "cable" of nerve fibers and tissues that runs through the hollowed centers of the stack of vertebrae forming the spine.

onco- mass, tumor, swelling

Examples:

- oncology (onco/logy)—the study of tumors
- oncolysis (onco/lysis)—the destruction of tumors and tumor cells
- oncogenesis (onco/gen/esis)—the production or causation of tumors

-oncus (-onc/us)—designation for a swelling or tumor:
- arthroncus (arthr/onc/us)—swelling of a joint
- blepharoncus (blephar/onc/us)—tumor on the eyelid
- cheiloncus (cheil/onc/us)—a tumor of the lip
- glossoncus (gloss/onc/us)—a swelling of the tongue
- mastoncus (mast/onc/us)—a tumor of the breast or mammary gland

onych- nail; claw / a fingernail, a toenail

Examples:

- onychectomy (onych/ectomy)—surgical removal of the nail or nail bed
- onychogenic (onych/gen/ic)—forming or producing nail substance
- onychia (onych/ia)—inflammation of the nail bed (matrix) resulting in loss of the nail, also called onychitis (onych/itis)

-onychium, -onychia (-onych/ium, -onych/ia)—suffixes used to indicate region(s) and conditions of the nail(s):
- eponychium (ep/onych/ium)—the cuticle; the narrow band of skin (epidermis) that extends from the nail wall into the nail surface
- leukonychia (leuk/onych/ia)—whitish spots or discoloration of the nails

or-   mouth / the mouth; the body structure bounded at the front by the lips and containing the tongue and teeth

This root is seen in the well-known word *oral* meaning "pertaining to the mouth."

Examples:
- orad (or/ad)—toward the mouth
- circumoral (circum/or/al)—the area around the mouth (*circum* means around as in circumference, the distance around a circle)

☞   **Note:** *Or-* is used to designate the mouth as an anatomical part; *stom-*, *stomat-* is used to designate disease, injuries and therapy on the mouth.

oto-   ear / the ear

Because the ear is such a prominent feature of the head, it is used not only for conditions that affect the ear, e.g. pain (ot/algia), water in the ear (hydr/ot/is), inflammation (ot/itis), but also as a landmark for use in locating other body parts that are less visible; this is indicated by the suffix stem *-otic* (-ot/ic) or *-otid* (-ot/id).

Examples:
- parotid (par/ot/id)—situated near the ear such as the parotid gland, a salivary gland located near the ear
- epiotic (epi/ot/ic)—situated on or above the ear
- entotic or endotic (ent/ot/ic or end/ot/ic)—situated in or arising in the ear

ovar-   egg (the female reproductive cell) / the paired female reproductive organ that produces eggs and female sex hormones✻ egg container

The root ov- means "egg" and forms the medical words:
- ovum (ov/um)—to denote the female reproductive cell that, upon fertilization after encountering semen- (see Lesson 4), begins the process of reproduction (the production of offspring)
- ova (ov/a)—"eggs," the plural of ovum

The combination of elements in ov/ar- literally means "place for the ova" or, more familiarly, "an egg container."

Examples:
- ovary (*ov/ar/y*)—name for the sexual gland in the female in which the ova are formed
- ovariogenic (ovari/o/gen/ic)—produced in or arising in the ovary
- ovariocentesis (ovari/o/centesis)—surgical puncture of an ovary

-pexy suspension; fixation / the surgical act of fastening or making firm or solid

When organs are displaced (-ptosis), the surgical operation to repair this condition by restoring the organ to its proper place is called "fixation" or "suspension." The suffix -*pexy* is used to denote this procedure and may be interpreted as "surgical fixation of."

Examples:
- nephropexy (nephr/o/pexy)—surgical fixation of the kidney
- gastropexy (gastr/o/pexy)—surgical fixation of the stomach
- hysteropexy (hyster/o/pexy)— surgical fixation of the womb

pyl-, pyloro- gate / a gate, an opening, a passage

These elements have a basic root *pyl-* that carries the meaning "gate" or "opening."

The root *pyle-* is used for relationships to an important vein, the portal vein, which is a large vein carrying blood from the digestive organs and the spleen to the liver:
- pylic (pyl/ic)—pertaining to the portal vein
- pylethrombosis (pyle/thromb/osis)—a condition of clotting in the portal vein (*thromb-* is an element taught in Lesson 11 and it means clot)

The root *pylor-* that literally means "gate keeper" is used for relationships to the pylorus which is the opening of the stomach into the intestines through which the stomach contents pass into the intestines:
- pyloric (pylor/ic)—pertaining to the pylorus
- gastropylor- (gastr/o/pylor)—form for the stomach and the pylorus
- gastropyloric (gastr/o/pylor/ic)—pertaining to the stomach and the pylorus
- gastropylorectomy (gastr/o/pylor/ectomy)—excision of the pyloric portion of the stomach

sphenic a wedge; wedge-shaped

Examples:
- sphenoid (sphen/oid)—resembling a wedge; in the shape of a wedge
- sphenoid bone (sphen/oid)—an irregular wedge-shaped bone at the base of the cranium
- sphenocephaly (sphen/o/cephal/y)—a developmental abnormality characterized by a wedge-shaped appearance of the head

spiro- coil / a coil- a winding, twisting

Examples:
- spiroid (spir/oid)—resembling a spiral or coil
- spiradeno- (spir/aden/o-)—a form used interchangeably with hidradeno-

(hidr/aden/o) to denote a sweat gland; so called because of the spiral shape of a sweat gland

Spiro- should not be confused with *spir-* appearing in words as perspire (per/spir/e), perspiration (per/spir/ation), aspiration (a/spir/ation), respiration (re/spir/ation). In these the element means "breath" or "breathing."

---

squam-   scaley a scale, a platelike structure (such as scales and scaly structure on a fish)

Examples:
- squama (squam/a)—a scale or platelike structure
- squamous, squamosa (squam/ous, squam/osa)—scaly or platelike
- squamate (squam/ate)—scaly; having or resembling scales

The rough skin which peels as a result of sunburn is an example of squama. Squamous carcinoma (also squamous cell carcinoma) is skin cancer.

---

sub-   under, beneath, below / less than

Examples:
- subdermal (sub/derm/al)—situated or occurring under the skin
- subnormal (sub/norm/al)— below or less than normal
- sublingual (sub/lingu/al)—located beneath the tongue; also subglossal
- subinflammation (sub/inflammation)—a slight or mild inflammation (sub = below, less than, slight or mild)
- submania (sub/man/ia)—mania of a moderate type; also hypomania

---

thorac-   chest / the part of the body situated between the neck and the abdomen and supported by the cagelike structure formed by the ribs

Examples:
- thorax—medical name for the chest; also called thorac/ic cavity
- thoracic (thorac/ic)—(sometimes thor/ac/al)—pertaining to the chest
- thoracogastr- (thorac/o/gastr-)—relating to the stomach and chest (thorax)
- thoracicoabdominal (thorac/ic/o/abdomin/al)—pertaining to the chest and the abdomen
- suprathoracic (supra/thorac/ic)—situated above the thorax
- hemothorax (hem/o/thorax)—a collection of blood in the lung cavity

---

vesic-   bladder / a bladder; the urinary bladder   fluid filled sack

Examples:
- vesica (vesic/a)—general term for a bladder
- vesical (vesic/al)—pertaining to (principally) the urinary bladder

- vesico- (vesic/o)—form relating to a bladder or the urinary bladder
- vesicle—medical name for a small bladder, sac or blister containing liquid
- vesicula (vesic/ul/a)—general term used in anatomical nomenclature for a vesicle (small sac or bladder)
- vesicular (vesic/ul/ar)—formed or constructed like a small sac or bladder; containing, made up of, or characterized by small saclike bodies

Vesic- compared with *cyst-*: again we have two roots that have the same meaning but are applied differently. *Vesic-* is the root generally used in naming the various bladders or bladder-like structures in the body; *cyst-* is the root generally used in naming of diseases and therapeutic procedures involving bladders or bladder-like structures.

viscero-   organ / an internal organ or the internal organs of the body especially those located in the large cavity of the trunk such as the heart, the liver, the intestines, etc.

Examples:
- visceral (viscer/al)—pertaining to an internal organ, especially those in the abdomen
- viscera (viscer/a)—name for internal organs taken collectively, especially those in the abdomen
- viscerad (viscer/ad)—toward the viscera
- visceroptosis (viscer/o/ptosis)—a dropping or falling down of the viscera due, for example, to the weakness of the abdominal muscles

Lesson 5—Element Recognition

Separate the word terminals, elements, and connecting vowels of the following medical terms from right to left by inserting a slash mark (/) between them.

Example: pylorogastrectomy—pyloro/gastr/ectomy

o v / i / g e n e s i s
the production of eggs

t h o r a c / e n t / e s i s
binding within the chest

o t / o / l i t h / i a s i s
condition of stones in the ear

b i l i / o u s
full of having bile

s q u a m / o u s
having scales or platelike structures

m e n i n g / o / c e r e b r / i t i s
inflammation of the brain membrane surrounding the brain & the brain

c e c / o / p e x y
fixed fixation of the pouch at the beginning of L intestine

m a c u l / a
a spot or blotch

n e p h r / o / p e x y
surgical fixation of the kidney

o n c / o / s i s
tumor condition

o r / a l o g y
study of the mouth

s u b / c o s t / a l
pertaining to under the ribs

m y e l / o / m a l a c i a
softening of bone marrow the spinal cord

s p i r / o i d
resembling a spiral or coil

l a c r i m / o t o m y
cutting into the tear duct for purpose of R.E.D

v i s c e r / o / p t o s i s
the dropping of an organ

l a c t i / g e n o u s
producing by milk

o n y c h / o / m a l a c i a
softening of the nails

t h o r a c / o / m y / o / d y n i a
pain in the chest muscles

p y l o r / o / s t e n / o / s i s
condition narrowing of the passage of the mouth

v e s i c / o / c e l e
hernia in the bladder through the vaginal wall

m y e l / o / m e n i n g / i t i s
inflammation of the membrane covering the brain and spinal cord

a n t i / m y c o / t i c
pertaining to opposing fungus

m y c o / m y r i n g / i t i s
inflammation of the eardrum due to fungus

o n c o l o g y
the study of tumors

s u b / g l o s s / i t i s
inflammation under the tongue

v i s c e r / a l g i a
pain in an organ

g a l a c t / o / c e l e
cystic tumor of breast caused by a blocked milk duct

o n y c h / o / r r h e x i s
rupture of a nail

t h o r a c / o / s c o p / y
to observe the chest

m y c / o / s i s
condition of fungus

a n t i / p l a s t / i c
pertaining to

h e p a t / o / p e x y
surgical fixation suspension of the liver

c e c / u m
large pouch at the beginning of the large intestine with only 1 opening

s p h e n / o i d / o t o m y
surgical incision of the wedge shaped bone of the skull for red

v e s i c / o t o m y
surgical incision of the bladder for purpose of red

o v / o i d
resembling an egg

a r t h r / o / c e n t / e s i s
binding surgical puncture of a joint to remove fluid

o t / o / d y n i a
pain in the ear

b i l i / g e n e s i s
production of bile

m e n i n g / e o / r r h a p h y
the suturing membrane covering the brain and spinal cord

s p h e n / o / c e p h a l / y
a developmental abnormality

- 100 -

Lesson 5—Interpretation Exercise

Complete the following statements by printing the meanings of the elements that make up the medical term in the proper blanks. (Remember, most medical terms are interpreted from right to left.)

5-1.   An antigen (anti/gen) is a substance when introduced into the body stimulates the

_____ of an opposing substance known as an antibody.

5-2.   The term biliary (bili/ary) denotes pertaining to or of the _____.

5-3.   The cecum (cec/um) is a large pouch, having only_____ opening, located at

the beginning of the large intestine.

5-4.   Arthrocentesis (arthr/o/centesis) refers to a surgical _____ of a

_____.

5-5.   Hallux is the medical name for the _____ _____.

5-6.   The lacrimal (lacrim/al) glands secrete _____.

5-7.   The term lacteal (lact/e/al) pertains to or of _____.

5-8.   A macula (macul/a) is a _____.

5-9.   Meningitis (mening/itis) is an _____ of the _____ covering the

brain and spinal cord.

5-10.   Mycosis (myc/osis) is a _____ of _____.

5-11.   Osteomyelitis (oste/o/myel/itis) is an _____ of a _____ and its

_____.

5-12.   Mastoncus (mast/onc/us) denotes a _____ of the _____ or

mammary gland.

5-13.   The term leukonychia (leuk/oncyh/ia) refers to _____ spots or discoloration of the _____.

5-14.   Circumoral (circum/or/al) refers to the area _____ the _____.

5-15.   The term parotid (par/ot/id) denotes being situated _____ the _____.

5-16.   Ovariogenic (ovari/o/gen/ic) refers to being _____ in the _____.

5-17.   Hysteropexy (hyster/o/pexy) is the surgical _____ of the _____.

5-18.   A gastropylorectomy (gastr/o/pylor/ectomy) is the surgical _____ of the portion of the _____ containing the _____ into the intestines.

5-19.   The term sphenic (sphen/ic) pertains to being _____ shaped.

5-20.   Spiroid (spir/oid) means _____ a _____.

5-21.   The term squamous (squam/ous) pertains to being _____.

5-22.   Sublingual (sub/lingu/al) pertains to being located _____ the _____.

5-23.   The term thoracicoabdominal (thorac/ic/o/abdomin/al) denotes pertaining to or of the _____ and the _____.

5-24.   Vesica (vesic/a) is a general term for a _____.

5-25.   A visceral (viscer/al) denotes pertaining to an internal _____ especially in the abdomen.

Lesson 6

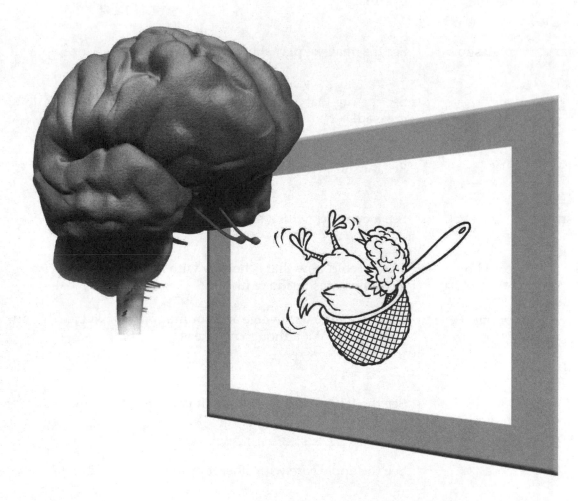

Lesson 6—Review

Element	Audionym	Visual Image	Meaning
✱ physio-	physics book	See the **physi**cs book with a **nature** boy streaking out of it!	~~nature~~ body
bucc(o)-	bucket	See the **buc**ket with **real cheeks** on it!	cheek
palpebr-	pile of people	See the **pile** of **pe**ople with gigantic **eyelids**!	eyelid
-plasia	play show	See the image of **play sh**ow **developing** film!	development
rug-	rug	See the **rug** that is **wrinkled, fold**ed, and **crease**d!	wrinkle, fold, crease
aur-	"R"	See the **"R"** with an **ear** on it!	ear
acoust(i)-	a cue stick	See **a cue sti**ck with a **hearing** aid on it!	hearing
colp(o)-	cold bow	See the **col**d **bo**w that is **hollow** with **Virginia** hams inside of it!	hollow, vagina
phon-	phone	See the **phone** with **voice** and **sound** coming out of it although no one is using it!	voice, sound
✱ leio-	lei	See the **lei** that has no flowers. It is **smooth**!	smooth
cor	core	See the apple **core** with a **heart** inside it!	heart
ren-	rain	See it **rain**ing **kid**s on their **knee**s!	kidney

Element	Audionym	Visual Image	Meaning
orchi-	orchid	See the **orchi**d with **tests** stuck in it!	testis
encephal-	hen sieve fall	See the h**en** in a **sieve fall**ing. It has a **brain** instead of a head!	brain
✳ thalam-	the lamb	See **the lam**b as the w**inner** of the **Chamber** of Commerce Contest!	inner chamber
✳ plexus	plexiglass	See the **plexi**glass with gigantic **braid**s coming out of it!	braid
cilia	ceiling	See the **ceil**ing with huge **eyelash**es all over it!	eyelash
✳ dendr-	den door	See the **den d**oor in the **tree** with many **branches**!	tree, branching
phleb-	flip (flip chart)	See the **flip** chart covered with **vein**s!	vein
pilo-	pile on	See the man **pil**ing **on hair** on another man's head!	hair
histo-	his toe	See **his toe** with **tissue**s coming out of it!	tissue
stoma-	stone	See the **sto**ne with a huge **mouth** on it!	mouth
tympan-	tin pan	See the **tin pan** with an **ear** and **drum** in it!	eardrum
umbilic-	a bill lick	See **a bill** being **lick**ed with a **naval** officer coming out of it!	navel
salpingo-	Sally Bingo	See **Sal**ly playing **Bingo** sitting in an inner **tube**!	tube

Lesson 6—Worksheet

Print the audionym and meaning of the elements in the proper blanks:

Element	Audionym	Meaning
physio-		
bucc(o)-		
palpebr-		
plasia-		
rug-		
aur-		
acoust(i)		
colp(o)-		
phon-		
leio-		
cor		
ren-		
orchi-		
encephal-		
thalam-		
plexus		
cilia		
dendr-		
phleb-		
pilo-		
histo-		
stoma-		
tympan-		
umbilic-		
salpingo-		

Lesson 6—Word Terminals

-ian   belonging to or having some relation to; one believing in or following

Examples:
- Christ/ian, Grec/ian, Ind/ian, Florid/ian, Pennsylvan/ian (same as *-an*, see Lesson 2)

-ism   an abnormal condition

This terminal is similar in meaning to *-osis.*

Examples:
- alcohol/ism, morphin/ism, melan/ism

-ite   a part of the body or bodily organ

Example:
- dendrite (dendr/ite)—a body part characterized by its appearance of branching

-itic   pertaining to or affected by inflammation

This terminal is a combination of *-itis* (Lesson 1) and *-ic* ("pertaining to", Reading Assignment, Lesson 1) and is used to refer to a condition of inflammation.

Examples:
- arthr/itic, gastr/itic, nephr/itic

-on   noun ending; used to form the name of a thing from the root

Example:
- en/cephal/on

Lesson 6—Reading Assignment

acoust(i)- hearing; sound

Examples:
- acoustic (acoust/ic)—pertaining to hearing
- acoustogram (acoust/o/gram)—the graphic tracing of the measures of sound such as decibel levels and frequency per second

Because of the familiarity of *acousti-* in words for sound, we have chosen to present the root in this form. However, the basic root meaning sound is *acous-* or *acus-*:
- -acusis (-acu/sis)—used to denote a condition of hearing (also *-acusia*)
- anacusis (an/acu/sis)— "condition of not hearing"; total deafness (*an-* means "not" and is discussed in Lesson 10)
- hemianacusia (hemi/an/acus/ia)—loss of hearing in one ear only

aur- ear

Examples:
- auricle (aur/i/cle)—the projecting part of the ear lying outside the head
- auricul- (aur/i/cul)—form denoting relationship to the ear or to an ear-shaped appendage of a chamber of the heart
- auriculocranial (aur/i/cul/o/crani/al)—pertaining to an ear and the cranium
- auris (aur/is)—the ear

The element *oto-*, ear, (Lesson 5) is the more widely used form for denoting conditions of the ear and the therapeutic procedures to correct such conditions.

bucc(o)- cheek

Examples:
- buccal (bucc/al)—pertaining to the cheek; directed toward the cheek
- buccally (bucc/al/ly)—toward the cheek

This root is used widely as a landmark or point of reference in locating other (usually less prominent) structures or features of other structures. For example, in dentistry the buccal surface of a tooth is the surface on the side toward the cheek:
- buccocervical (bucc/o/cervic/al)—that surface of a tooth along its neckline (the part of the tooth at the point where it enters the gum) on the cheek side
- suprabuccal (supra/bucc/al)—above the cheek region

cilia eyelash / the lashes of the eye; also a hairlike projection

Examples:
- ciliary (cili/ary)—pertaining to the eyelashes; resembling the eyelashes

- cilium (cili/um)—the eyelashes; also sometimes the eyelid or the outer edge of the eyelid or the edge of the eyelid from which the eyelashes extend
- supercilia (super/cilia)—the eyebrows (*super-* is a prefix that is close in meaning to *supra-* [Lesson 3]; here it means "above"). Literally, then, the meaning is "above the eyelashes."
- ciliogenesis (cili/o/gen/esis)—the formation or development of cilia

colp(o)-   hollow; vagina / the canal in the female that forms a passage from the uterus to the outside of the body

pyo-pus

-colpos (-colp/os)—suffix stem used to denote a vaginal disorder of a specific type.

Examples:
- pyocolpos (py/o/colp/os)—collection of pus within the vagina
- hematocolpos (hemat/o/colp/os)—an accumulation of menstrual blood in the vagina
- colpitis (colp/itis)— inflammation of the vagina

☞   **Note:** *Vagin-* is also a root used to denote relationships to any sheathlike structure, but especially the vagina as defined above.
vaginal (vagin/al)—pertaining to the vagina; of the nature of a sheath

cor   heart / the heart / the muscular organ that maintains the circulation of the blood

This is a word used in international nomenclature to denote the heart. It is introduced to mark a distinction from the element *coron-* meaning "crown" that is often used broadly to indicate the heart and *cardi-* that is the most widely used root to name conditions of the heart and therapeutic procedures applied to the heart.

Another form in which *cor* appears is *cord-* in such words as:
- cordate (cord/ate)—heart-shaped
- cordial (cord/i/al)—stimulating the heart

✱ *dendr-*   tree; branching (as in the nervous system)

This descriptive root that can be interpreted as "branching" is used to describe body structures or parts resembling the branching of a tree; especially used for the nerve fibers that extend from a nerve cell (dendrite).

Examples:
- dendrite (dendr/ite)—name for the nerve fibers that extend from a nerve cell
- dendritic (dendr/it/ic)—resembling a dendrite; branching like a tree
- dendroid (dendr/oid)—branching like a tree

encephal- brain

> Examples:
> - encephalic (en/cephal/ic)—pertaining to the brain; also, lying within the cranial cavity
> - encephalon (en/cephal/on)—name for the brain
>
> The element *cephal* was introduced in Lesson 3; however, because of the frequent use of *encephal-* in medical terminology, we have introduced *encephal-* as an element in order that you might more easily remember the "brain" meaning of *encephal-*.

histo- tissue / a mass of cells that forms one of the structural materials out of which the body is built up; a weblike structure

> Examples:
> An important clue for recognizing words dealing with tissues is the word ending *-ium* (sometimes *eum*). Many (probably most) of the words you encounter having an *-ium* (or *-eum*) ending denote tissues:
> - endocardium (end/o/card/ium)—the tissue (membrane) lining the heart
> - endosteum (end/ost/eum)—the tissue lining the cavity of a bone and surrounding the bone marrow
> - histocyte (hist/o/cyt/e)—a tissue cell
> - histoma (hist/oma)—a tumor formed from fully developed tissue such as blood vessels, muscles, etc.
> - histolysis (hist/o/lysis)—the breaking down and destruction of tissue
> - histology (hist/ology)—the study (usually microscopic) of the structure, composition and functions of the tissues

✳*leio-* smooth / especially, the "smooth" or "involuntary" muscles

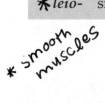
* smooth muscles

> This descriptive root may be used in reference to any smooth surface; it is especially used in the description of tumors to distinguish the so called "smooth" muscles that are generally found in the walls of the stomach, intestines, vessels and glands; they are also in the very small muscles of the skin and, when contracted, produce what is called "goose flesh." The "smooth muscles" are also called "involuntary muscles" because they are not under control of the will.
>
> Examples:
> - leiomyoma (leio/my/oma)—a tumor composed of smooth muscle fibers
> - leiodermia (leio/derm/ia)—abnormal glossiness or smoothness of the skin

orchi- testis / testicle; one of the two male reproductive glands

testis = 1
testes = 2

> Examples:
> - orchic, orchidic (orch/ic, orchid/ic)—pertaining to the testicles

- -orchidism, -orchism (-orchid/ism, -orch/ism)—a (specified) form or condition of the testes
- orchitis (orch/itis)—inflammation of a testicle
- orchidopexy (orchid/o/pexy)—the surgical fixing in place of a displaced testicle

---

palpebr- eyelid

LAD SNOR

Examples:
- palpebral (palpebr/al)—pertaining to an eyelid
- palpebra (palpebr/a)—the eyelid
- palpebrate (palpebr/ate)—to wink
- palpebration (palpebr/ation)—abnormally frequent winking

Here is another root meaning "eyelid." The tendency to use *palpebr-* as the root for naming or referring to the eyelid as an anatomical part; *blephar-* is the root used principally for the naming of conditions and therapeutic procedures involving the eyelid.

---

phleb- vein / one of the branching blood vessels that carries blood toward the heart (compared to arteries which carry blood away from the heart)

Examples:
- phlebectasis (phleb/ectasis)—an enlargement (dilatation) of a vein; also phlebectasia
- phlebolith (phleb/o/lith)—"vein stone"; a bloodclot, in a vein, which has turned chalky
- phlebostenosis (phleb/o/sten/osis)—narrowing or constriction of a vein
- phlebophlebostomy (phleb/o/phleb/ostomy)—surgical openings to provide communication between two veins
- phlebitis (phleb/itis)—inflammation of a vein

---

phon- voice; sound

This description root is generally used to denote speech or body sounds; the body sounds may be those arising within the body (heart beats) or created by such means as percussion (tapping).

Examples:
- phonic, phonal (phon/ic, phon/al)—pertaining to the voice
- phonocardiogram (phon/o/cardi/o/gram)—a record of heart sounds
- phonogram (phon/o/gram)—a record of any sound
- phonomyogram (phon/o/my/o/gram)—a record of the sound produced by muscle action
- phonopathy (phon/o/path/y)—any disease or disorder of the organs of speech

physio- ᴧᴧᴧᴧ / the body (frequently as opposed to the mind)

Examples:
- physiology (physi/ology)—the study of the functions of the body and its parts
  - pathologic physiology (path/o/log/ic physi/ology)—the study of disordered function or of function in diseased tissue
  - general physiology (physi/ology)—the study of the general laws of life and functional activity
- physiatrics (phys/iatr/ics)—the diagnosis and treatment of disease with the aid of physical agents such as light, heat, cold, water, and electricity, or with mechanical apparatus
- physician (phys/ic/ian)—an authorized practitioner of medicine
  - attending physician (phys/ic/ian)—a physician who attends a hospital at stated times to visit the patients and give direction as to their treatment
  - resident physician (phys/ic/ian)—a graduate and licensed physician resident in a hospital

pilo- hair

Examples:
- pilus (pil/us)—a hair
- pilous, pilose , pileous, pilosity (pil/ous, pil/ose, pil/eous, pil/os/ity)—hairiness, covered with hair
- pilosis (pil/osis)—excessive growth of hair
- pilocystic (pil/o/cyst/ic)—cystlike and containing hair; used to describe certain skin tumors
- depilation (de/pil/ation)— the process of removing hair; the agent for hair removal is a de/pil/atory (the prefix de- has a meaning "remove" as in the familiar words de/hydr/ate, de/magnetize, de/contaminate, etc.)

-plasia development or growth

plasm

Examples:
- hyperplasia (hyper/plasia)—abnormal increase in growth; usually applied to abnormal increase in the cells making up tissues
- hypoplasia (hypo/plasia)—incomplete or defective development
- mastoplasia (mast/o/plasia)—the development of breast tissue

✱ ***plexus*** ᴧᴧᴧᴧ, an <u>interweaving</u> or <u>network</u> / a network or <u>tangle</u> used in medical (anatomical) terminology to designate a network of Lymphatic vessels, nerves or veins

Examples:
- plexal (plex/al)—pertaining to a plexus
- plexiform (plex/i/form)—resembling a plexus or network
- subplexal (sub/plex/al)—situated beneath a plexus or network of vessels, nerves or veins

ren- kidneys / a kidney; either of a pair of glandular organs in the lower back that filter water and waste from the blood and secrete them as urine (also *nephr-*)

Example:
- renal (ren/al)—pertaining to the kidney

The root *ren-* is used principally as a landmark, that is, a point of reference in locating other nearby structures:
- supraren- (supra/ren-)—situated above the kidney, especially with reference to the suprarenal gland

The root *nephr-* is used principally to name the conditions affecting the kidneys (diseases, symptoms, etc.) and the surgical procedures performed on the kidneys.
- nephrectomy (nephr/ectomy)—surgical removal of a kidney

rug- wrinkle; fold; crease

Examples: rugae=2
- ruga (rug/a)—=1 a ridge, wrinkle or fold, as of mucous membrane
- rugose, rugous (rug/ose, rug/ous)—characterized by wrinkles
- rugosity (rug/osity)—the condition of being wrinkled; a fold, ridge or wrinkle

salpingo- tube / any tube or trumpet-shaped structure, especially the uterine tube into which the ovum (egg cell) passes when it leaves the ovary (egg case); also the auditory (hearing) tube

The root *salping-* might better be remembered as tuba-like since, like a tuba, it is a tube which is flared at the end. The name for such a tube (or tuba-like) structure is salpinx. There are two important structures in the body having this shape:

The fallopian tubes (also called uterine tubes): two tubes in the reproductive system of the female which transmit the ovum (eggs) to the uterus (womb) and in that fertilization (conception) begins.

The Eustachian Tube: tube in the ear that extends from the ear to the throat and is the means of equalizing pressure within the inner ear with the pressure of the atmosphere. When pressure builds on the tympanic membrane (changes in altitude such as airplane and elevator ascents and descents), relief is obtained by equalizing this pressure by yawning, swallowing, or noseblowing that relieves the pressure difference in the eustachian tube. Also called the hearing tube and auditory tube.

Examples:
- salpingostomy (salping/ostomy)—the making (by surgery) of an opening into the fallopian (uterine) tube because the natural opening has become closed
- endosalpinx (end/o/salpin/x)—the mucous membrane lining the salpinx (the fallopian or uterine tube)

stoma-   mouth or opening / the mouth of the face

In Lesson 2, you learned the root *stoma-* in the form *-ostomy,* a mouthlike opening that is derived from "stoma".

The root may appear in the form *stomat-*:

- stomatology (stomat/ology)—the branch of medicine that treats the mouth and its diseases
- stomatoplasty (stomat/o/plast/y)—plastic surgery of, operative repair of, defects of the mouth
- stomatogastric (stomat/o/gastr/ic)—pertaining to the stomach and the mouth
- stomatalgia (stomat/algia)—"mouth pain"; pain in the mouth; also stom/algia

✳ **thalam-**   ~~inner chamber~~ / large gray mass that is part of the brain or

switchboard of the brain

Examples:

- thalamus (thalam/us)—name for the large gray mass in the brain
- thalamic (thalam/ic)— pertaining to the thalamus

This root is used in medical terminology to show relations to the thalamus, the part of the brain which serves as a "switchboard" for the relaying of "messages." It is in this section that sensations such as pain, smell, touch are correlated with the taking of actions.

The root is used principally as a landmark. The thalam/us, epi/thalam/us, hypo/thalam/us, and sub/ thalam/us are terms applied to name the parts (chambers) of a large brain cavity called the di/en/ cephal/on (*di-* is a prefix meaning "two").

tympan-   eardrum or its enclosure

Examples:

- tympanum (tympan/um)—name for the enclosure or chamber in which the eardrum is located; also called the tympanic cavity
- tympanic membrane (tympan/ic)—name for the eardrum
- tympanal (tympan/al)—pertaining to the tympanum (the tympanic cavity); pertaining to the tympanic cavity (the eardrum)
- tympanic (tympan/ic)—pertaining to the tympanum (the tympanic cavity)

umbilic-   navel / "belly button"

Examples:

- umbilicus (umbilic/us)—name for the navel ("belly button")
- umbilical (umbilic/al)—pertaining to the umbilicus or navel
- umbilicectomy (umbilic/ectomy)—excision of the umbilicus
- parumbilical (par/umbilic/al)—near the navel

Lesson 6—Element Recognition

Separate the word terminals, elements, and connecting vowels of the following medical terms from right to left by inserting a slash mark (/) between them.

Example: encephalomyelitis—en/cephal/o/myel/itis

physi/o/lysis
destruction of the body *~~~~~*

bucco/gingiv/al
pertaining to the gums & cheek

palpebr/itis
inflammation of the eyelid

colp/o/hyper/plasia
over growth of the vagina

auri/scope
instrument used to observe the ear

acoust/ic
pertaining to hearing

colp/o/celio/centesis
puncture of the abdomen to get to the vagina

phon/o/cardi/o/gram
a record of heart sounds

leio/my/oma
tumor composed of smooth muscle fibers

ren/o/troph/ic
development of the kidneys

orchid/optosis
condition of dropping testes

encephal/o/malacia
softening of the brain

cili/o/genesis
production of eyelashes hair like structures

dendr/oid
branching like a tree

phlebo/lith/iasis
condition of stones in the vein

pil/o/sis
excessive growth of hair

hist/oid
tissue like

stomat/o/plast/y
surgical repair of defects of the mouth

tympan/ectomy
surgical removal of all or part of the eardrum

salping/ostomy
creat an opening in the fallopian tubes

leio/derm/ia
condition of smooth skin

ren/i/cardi/ac
pertaining to heart & kidneys

orchi/o/myel/oma
tumor composed of marrow in the testes

encephal/o/lith
stones in the brain

cili/ectomy
surgical removal of all or part of me eyelashes hair like projection

phleb/o/rrhexis
rupturing of a vein

pil/o/logy
the study of hair

hist/o/lysis
destruction of tissue

stomat/o/malacia
softening of the mouth

tympan/o/tomy
cutting into the eardrum for purpose of R.E.D.

umbil/ectomy
surgical removal of all or part of the belly button

salping/o/cele
hernia of the fallopian tube

physi/o/logy
study of the body & its functions

bucco/lingual
pertaining to the tongue & cheek

palpebr/al
pertaining to the eyelid

hypo/plasia less than normal
incomplete or defective development

colp/ectasis
expansion or stretching of the vagina

phon/o/path/y
disease of the organs of speech

stomat/algia
pain in the mouth

salping/itis
inflammation of the fallopian tubes

hist/o/ma
a tumor formed from fully developed tissue

colp/o/rrhaphy
suturing of the vagina

- 115 -

Lesson 6—Interpretation Exercise

Complete the following statements by printing the meanings of the elements that make up the medical term in the proper blanks. (Remember, most medical terms are interpreted from right to left.)

6-1.   Acoustic (acoust/ic) is a term that denotes pertaining to _____.

6-2.   The term auriculocranial (aur/i/cul/o/crani/al) pertains to the _____ and the _____.

6-3.   Suprabuccal (supra/bucc/al) refers to _____ the _____.

6-4.   The term ciliary (cili/ary) denotes pertaining to or resembling the _____.

6-5.   Colpitis (colp/itis) is an _____ of the _____.

6-6.   Cor is a word used internationally to denote the _____.

6-7.   Dendroid (dendr/oid) denotes _____ a _____.

6-8.   Encephalitis (en/cephal/itis)is an _____ of the _____.

6-9.   A histocyte (hist/o/cyt/e) is a _____ _____.

6-10.   A leiomyoma (leio/my/oma) is a _____ comprised of _____ _____ fibers.

6-11.   Orchidopexy (orchid/o/pexy) is the surgical _____ of a displaced _____.

6-12.   Palpebra (palpebr/a) is the medical name for the _____.

6-13   Phlebostenosis (phleb/o/sten/osis) is a _____ of a _____.

6-14. A phonocardiogram (phon/o/cardi/o/gram) is a _____ of _____ sounds.

6-15. Physiology (physi/ology) is the _____ of the _____ and its parts.

6-16. The term pilocystic (pil/o/cyst/ic) pertains to being _____-like and containing _____.

6-17. Mastoplasia (mast/o/plasia) refers to the _____ of _____ tissue.

6-18. The term subplexal (sub/plex/al) denotes being _____ the plexus which is a _____of vessels, nerves or veins.

6-19. The term suprarenal (supra/ren/al) refers to being situated _____ the _____.

6-20. The term rugous (rug/ous) denotes being characterized by_____.

6-21. A salpingostomy (salping/ostomy) is the surgical procedure of making an _____ into the fallopian _____.

6-22. The term stomatalgia (stomat/algia) refers to _____ in the _____.

6-23. The root thalam- means _____ _____ and is used to show relationship to the thalamus which is the large grey mass of the brain.

6-24. The tympanum (tympan/um) is the name of the enclosure in which the_____ is located.

6-25. The term parumbilical (par/umbilic/al) refers to being near the _____.

Lesson 7

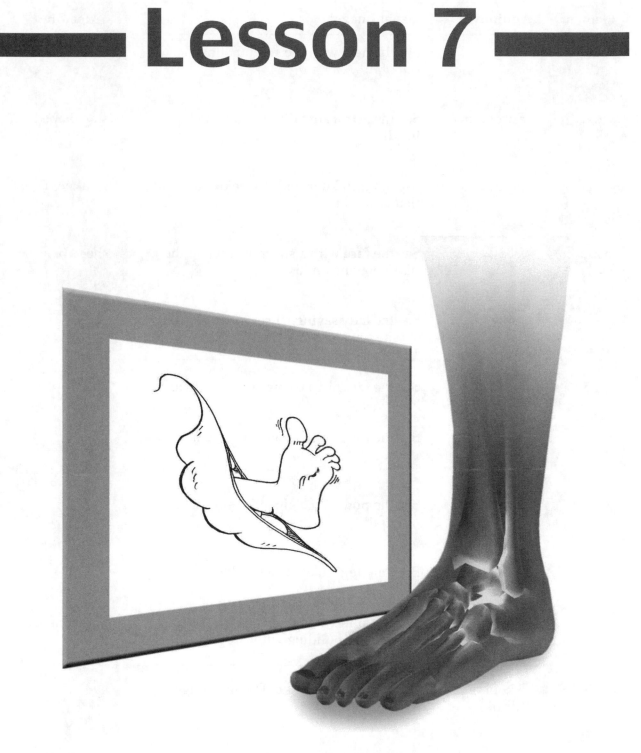

Lesson 7—Review

Element	Audionym	Visual Image	Meaning
helio-	heel	See the **heel** with the **sun** bursting out of it!	sun
astr-	astronaut	See the **astr**onaut with the **star shaped** head!	star shaped
*-asthenia	his thin knee	See **his thin knee** with a **week**ly calendar tied around it!	weakness
fascia	face	See the **face** with a **sheet** over it and the **band** playing on it!	sheet, band
iso-	I sew	See the lady saying, "**I sew** with **a quail**" as she sews with the quail!	equal
tarso-	tar	See the **tar** with a tri**angle** stuck into it!	ankle
-tope	top	See the **top** spinning with a **place**mat on it!	place
pod-	pod	See the **pod** with a gigantic **foot** sticking out of it!	foot
*malign-	my leg	See "**my leg**" made of a baseball **bat**!	bad
*adnexa-	annex	See the **annex tie**d or connected to the main building with a rope!	ties, connection
ocul-	a kool (drink)	See the image of "**a kool**" with a huge **eye** on it!	eye
lapar-	lap	See the **lap** holding an **apple** and a **wall**!	abdominal wall

Lesson 7—Review

Element	Audionym	Visual Image	Meaning
dacry-	daiquiri (drink)	See the **daiquiri cry**ing a gigantic **tear**!	tear
ment-	mint	See the two people pulling and fighting over the **mint** saying, "**Mine! Mine!**"!	mind
part-	part	See the **part** in the hair with a **labor**er **bring**ing **forth** a two by **four**!	labor, bring forth
✱ scler(a)-	scholar	See the **scholar** wearing a **hard** hat!	hard
somato-	sew my toe	See the man saying, 'I **sew my toe** onto my **body**"!	body
✱ trachel-	tray coal	See the **tray** of **coal** with a **neck** sticking out of it!	neck
sinus	sign us	See the baseball players saying, "**sign us** in this **hollow space**"!	hollow space
hypno-	hypnotist	See the **hypno**tist putting himself to **sleep**!	sleep
✱ sept-	sipped	See the person **sip**ping a drink through a **wall** with a **fence** on it!	wall, fence
✱ scirr(h)-	skirt	See the **skirt** with **hard** hats all over it!	hard
antr-	ant tree	See the **ant** in a **tree** falling into a gigantic **cave-in**!	cavity
-crine	cry'n	See the person **cry'n to see** the **crate**!	to secrete
✱ dura	door	See the **door** with **hard** hats all over it!	hard

- 121 -

Lesson 7—Worksheet

Print the audionym and meaning of the elements in the proper blanks:

Element	Audionym	Meaning
helio-		
astr-		
-asthenia		
fascia		
iso-		
tarso-		
-tope		
pod-		
malign-		
adnexa-		
ocul-		
lapar-		
dacry-		
ment-		
part-		
scler(a)-		
somato-		
trachel-		
sinus		
hypno-		
sept-		
scirr(h)-		
antr-		
-crine		
dura		

Lesson 7—Word Terminals

-ance, -ancy	a state or condition; the act of

Examples:
- brilliance (brilli/ance)—the state or condition of being brilliant
- elegance (eleg/ance)—the state or condition of being elegant
- assistance (assist/ance)—the act of assisting
- resistance (resist/ance)—the act of resisting

-ition	(same meaning as *-ation*, see Word Terminals, Lesson 4) a process, action or condition

Examples:
- addition (add/ition)—the process of adding
- prohibition (prohib/ition)—the act of denying, prohibiting
- ambition (amb/ition)—a state of striving for achievement

-ician	of or belonging to; frequently, a person belonging to or associated with

This terminal is a combination of *-ic* (Word Terminals, Lesson 1) and *-ian* (see *-an, -ian*, Word Terminals, Lesson 2) and carries the same meaning as *-an, -ian*

Examples:
- techn/ician, electr/ician, phys/ician, mathemat/ician

a, an, a d, de, pre, post

Lesson 7—Reading Assignment

adnexa ~~ties; connections~~ / appendages or adjacent parts

This word is a combination of a prefix *ad-* meaning "to" plus the root *nex-* meaning "join." Literally, the word means "joined to" and is applied chiefly to refer to the ocular adnexa, the appendages to the eye such as the lacrimal apparatus and the uterine adnexa, the appendages or adjacent parts to the womb such as the ovaries, the uterine tubes and the ligaments.

Examples:
- adnexopexy (adnex/o/pexy)—the operation of fixing the uterine adnexa to the abdominal walls
- adnexitis (adnex/itis)—inflammation of the uterine adnexa

antr- ~~cavity or chamber~~ / a sinus; a hollow space; ~~a cavity~~

Examples:
- antrum (antr/um)—a sinus; a cavity or chamber, especially within a bone
- antral (antr/al)—pertaining to a sinus or an antrum

The words antrum and sinus are synonyms in most applications. Generally, *sinus* is used to name a cavity or chamber as, for example, nasal sinus or nasal sinuses. *Antr-* is more frequently used as a root in forming single words relating to sinuses or antrums.

Examples:
- antrostomy (antr/ostomy)—the operation of making an opening into an antrum for the purpose of drainage
- antrodynia (antr/odyn/ia)—pain in an antrum

-asthenia weakness / lack of strength, "not strong"

This suffix combination is formed from three useful elements, the prefix *a-* meaning "not" or "lacking" plus the root *sthen-* meaning "strength" or "strong" plus the word ending *-ia* meaning "morbid (diseased) condition." Literally, the combination can be translated as "a condition of lacking strength" or "weakness."

Preceeding elements are added to provide more information, such as:
- adenasthenia (aden/ asthenia)—a weakness in glandular secretion; deficient glandular activity
- gastric adenasthenia (gastr/ic aden/asthenia)—deficient glandular secretion in the stomach

Asthen- may also be used with the same meaning "lacking strength" or "weakness:"
- asthenia (asthen/ia)—lack or loss of strength and energy; weakness

- 124 -

- asthenic (asthen/ic)—pertaining to or characterized by asthenia
- asthenopia (asthen/op/ia)—a condition of weakness in the eye

---

astr- star-shaped / resembling a star in form

Examples:

- astrocyte (astr/o/cyt/e)—a star-shaped cell, especially such a cell of the supporting structure of nervous tissue
- astroid (astr/oid)—star-shaped
- astrocytoma (astr/o/cyt/oma)—a tumor composed of star-shaped cells (astrocytes)

-crine to secrete

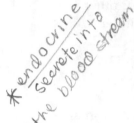
*endocrine
secrete into
the blood stream*

Examples:

- hypocrinia, also called hypocrinism (hypo/crin/ia, hypo/crin/ism)—deficient secretion of any endocrine gland
- hypercrinia, also called hypercrinism (hyper/crin/ia, hyper/crin/ism)—excessive secretion of any endocrine gland
- crinogenic (crin/o/gen/ic)—stimulating (producing) secretion

This word ending, which is used to indicate secretions of body fluids, is most prominent in medical terminology in naming the endocrine system, the "secreting into" system. The endocrine system is made up of the endocrine glands which secrete the chemical substance hormone, into the blood stream. The endocrine system, in conjunction with the nervous system, carries on the activities of the body. Some of the endocrine glands and the functions they perform are:

thyroid gland—growth and metabolism
pituitary gland—skeletal growth
adrenal gland—responds to need for increased body activity under stress
gonads, the female ovaries and the male testes—reproduction

---

dacry- tear / tear of the eye

In Lesson 5, we learned that *lacrim-* is a root also meaning tear or tears of the eye. The root *lacrim-* is generally used to denote the body parts or structures having to do with the production of tears. Conditions relating to tear production are generally denoted by the root *dacry-*. Some illustrations will make the distinction clearer:

- dacryoadenitis (dacry/o/aden/itis)—inflammation of a lacrimal gland (a tear gland)
- dacryocystectomy (dacry/o/cyst/ectomy)—excision of the wall of the lacrimal sac

Note the relationships:

tear gland = lacrimal gland = dacryadeno-
tear sac or tear bladder = lacrimal sac = dacrycysto-

dura   ~~hard~~ / used principally as a shortened form of dura mater, the outermost, toughest and most fibrous of the three membranes (meninges) covering the brain and spinal cord

hardest of the meninges

Examples:

- dura mater (or dura)—the outermost of the three membranes covering the brain and spinal cord
- induration (in/dur/ation)—hardness; the act or process of becoming hard (*in-* has the ordinary sense of "within," thus induration has the literal meaning of "a process of within or inner hardness")
- superdural (super/dur/al)—situated above or external to the dura mater

fascia   ~~sheet; band~~ / a sheet or band of fibrous tissue

The name fascia is used to denote connective tissues that exist extensively throughout the body and serve the purpose of forming an outer layer for other tissues such as ligaments and tendons; fascia also serve as anchors or binders to support or hold other tissue structures such as muscle bundles which are held together and kept in place during movement by a sheathlike covering of fascia.

Examples:
- fasciculus (fasci/cul/us)—a small bundle or cluster; used to designate a small bundle of nerve or muscle fibers
- fasciodesis (fasci/o/desis)—the operation of suturing a fascia to one of the tissues attached to the skeleton
- fasciorrhaphy (fasci/o/rrhaphy)—the suturing together of torn fascia

helio-   sun; light / sunlight

This root is used principally to designate effects of the rays of the sun as in:
- heliosensitivity (helio/sensitivity)—sensitivity to sunlight
- heliosis (helio/sis)—sunstroke
- heliotherapy (helio/therapy)—the treatment of disease by exposing the body to the sun's rays; therapeutic sunbathing

hypno-   sleep

Examples:
- hypnotic (hypnot/ic)—inducing sleep; a drug that acts to induce sleep; pertaining to or of the nature of hypnotism
- hypnotism (hypnot/ism)—the method or practice of an artificially induced passive state in which there is increased responsiveness to suggestions and commands
- ahypnia (a/hypn/ia)—"not sleep" (You will recall that the prefix *a-* has a meaning "not."); abnormal wakefulness; insomnia

iso- equal / alike; the same

This prefix is used widely to indicate "sameness" as in:
- isocellular (iso/ cell/ul/ar)—composed of cells of the same size and kind
- isopia (is/op/ ia)—equality of vision in the two eyes

The prefix *iso-* can also be combined with the prefix *an-* meaning "not," to indicate "not equal" or "inequality":
- anisodont (an/is/odont)—having teeth of unequal size or length
- anisopia (an/is/op/ia)— inequality of vision in the two eyes
- anisomastia (an/iso/mast/ia)—inequality of the breasts

lapar- abdominal wall / loin (the part of the back between the end of the ribs and the hip), flank (the part of the side between the ribs and the hip)

Technically the root *lapar-* applies to the lower back and sides, that is, the soft fleshy parts of the back and sides between the bones of the ribs and the hip bone. However, the root is used loosely to include the front of the cavity as well. It is in this looser or wider sense that the frequent word laparotomy is used:
- laparotomy (lapar/otomy)—surgical incision of the flank; less correctly but more generally, abdominal incision at any point in the abdominal wall
- hysterolaparotomy (hyster/o/lapar/otomy)—incision of the womb through the abdominal wall
- thoracolaparotomy (thorac/o/lapar/otomy)—incision through both the thorax and the abdomen
- laparorrhaphy (lapar/o/rrhaphy)—suturing of the abdominal wall
- laparogastrostomy (lapar/o/ gastr/ostomy)—the creation of a permanent opening to the stomach through the abdominal wall

malign- bad; harmful / the tendency to progressively get worse *cancerous*

This root is derived from the Latin word "malignans" that means acting maliciously. It is used most always to denote something bad that is going to get worse:
- malignant (malign/ant)—tending to become progressively worse and to result in death if not treated
- malignancy (malign/ancy)—a tendency to spread or become progressively worse; used most frequently with cancerous growths which tend to progressively invade (spread among) the tissues of the body

Malignant and benign (Lesson 4) are opposites.

ment- the mind

Examples:
- mental (ment/al)—pertaining to the mind
- mentality (ment/al/ity)—mental power or activity

- dementia (de/ment/ia)—a general term for mental deterioration (the prefix *de-* means "down," "down from")

The root *ment-* meaning "mind" is not extensively used in forming medical terms, the root *psych-* being the preferred element in words or expressions relating to the mind. Also, there may be confusion with the more widely used root *ment-* meaning "chin."

ocul-   eye

Examples:
- ocular (ocul/ar)—pertaining to the eye
- oculus (ocul/us)—name for the eye
- oculonasal (ocul/o/nas/al)—pertaining to the eye and the nose
- oculopathy (ocul/o/path/y)—any disease or disorder of the eye

In Lesson 2 you learned the root *ophthalm-* also denotes the eye or eyes and that *opt-* is a form meaning visible, or denoting relationship to vision or sight. Both *ocul-* and *ophthalm-* relate to the eye as a physical or anatomical organ. *Ocul-* is generally used more as a landmark while *ophthalm-* is used more to designate conditions of the eye and therapies applied to it:

- oculofacial (ocul/o/facial)—pertaining to the eyes and face
- ophthalmorrhexis (ophthalm/o/rrhexis)—rupture of the eye or eyeball
- optician (opt/ic/ian)—one who prepares lens per a prescription to improve or correct vision

part-   labor; bring forth / bear / giving birth; delivery

This root is closely related to our common use of the word *part* in the sense of "to separate from" since delivery or giving birth is the process whereby the mother is separated or "parted" from her offspring.

Examples:
- parturition (part/ur/ition)—the act or process of giving birth to a child
- postpartum (post/part/um)—occurring after childbirth or after delivery
  post- means "after" and is discussed more fully in Lesson 10
- prepartal (pre/part/al)—occurring before or just previous to labor
  pre- means "before" and is discussed more fully in Lesson 10

Peri-around

pod-   foot

ped- foot

Examples:
- podalic (pod/al/ic)—accomplished by means of the foot, as in obstetrical deliveries (versions)
- -podia (-pod/ia)—condition of the foot

There is a related root _ped-_ that may denote either <u>foot</u> or <u>child</u>:
- pedodontics (ped/odont/ics)—the department of dentistry dealing with the oral health of children
- pedopathy (ped/o/path/y)—any disease of the foot
- pediatrician (ped/iatr/ician)—a physician specializing in the diseases of children

Examples:
- podiatry (pod/iatr/y)—the diagnosis and treatment of diseases of the foot
- podiatrist (pod/iatr/ist)—one who practices podiatry. Usually, a podiatrist is not a doctor of medicine and is limited by his license to diseases of the foot.

scirr(h)-   hard / relating to a hard tumor   _hard cancerous tumor_

The root _scirr-_ (frequently _scirrh-_) is used to denote relationships to a scirrhus which is the name for a hard, cancerous tumor.

Examples:
- scirrhus (scirrh/us)—name for a hard, cancerous tumor
- scirrhous (scirrh/ous)—pertaining to or of the nature of a scirrhus

-scirrhus is also used as a word ending, the first element(s) in the word adding additional description:
- mastoscirrhus (mast/o/scirrh/us)—a hard cancer of the breast
- dacryadenoscirrhus (dacry/aden/o/scirrh/us)—a hard cancerous tumor (a scirrhus) of the lacrimal (tear) gland

scler(a)   hard / hardness; also "the white of the eye"

Since the presence of hardness in body parts that are normally lacking in hardness is a frequent sign of a morbid (diseased) condition, the root _scler-_ is widely used in medical terms to indicate the condition of abnormal hardness:
- sclerous (scler/ous)—hard; indurated (in/dur/ated)
- sclerosis (scler/osis)—a hardening; an induration; especially hardening of a part from inflammation. It may also be used as a word ending (_-sclerosis_) with preceeding element(s) in the word providing more information.

Another frequent use of the element _scler-_ is in reference to the sclera, "the white of the eye," the white cover of the eyeball that surrounds the back five-sixths of the eyeball (The front one-sixth of this cover is called the cornea and will be discussed in Lesson 8):
- sclera (scler/a)—the tough, white supporting cover of the eyeball covering approximately the back five-sixths of its surface
- sclerotic (sclerot/ic)—pertaining to hardness or hardening; pertaining to the sclera

Usages of *dura, scirrh-, scler-:*

In this lesson we have presented three elements all of which carry a meaning of "hardness." Following is a clarifying summary:

> *Dura* is used principally as a shortened name for the *dura mater,* the hard outer covering of the brain and spinal cord. An important exception to this usage is the word induration (in/dur/ation) that means "hardness"or "the process of hardening."

> *Scirrh-* is used almost exclusively in reference to a hard, cancerous tumor.

> *Scler-* can mean "hardness" or be a reference to "the white of the eye."

---

sept-   wall; fence / a dividing wall or membrane

in fection

Examples:

- septum (sept/um)—a general term in anatomy to designate a dividing wall or partition
- nasal septum (nas/al sept/um)—the partition separating the two nasal cavities (nostrils)

When *sept-* is used with no other qualification as in septectomy (sept/ectomy), septotomy (sept/otomy), the reference is to the nasal septum:

- septal (sept/al)—pertaining to a septum
- septulum (septul/um)—a small separating wall or partition

---

sinus   hollow space / cavity; hollow; recess

in your skull

There are many cavities, hollows and spaces in the body that are designated as sinuses. The most familiar are the para/nasal sinuses that are air cavities in the cranial bones communicating with the nasal cavity.

Examples:

- sinusoid (sinus/oid)—resembling a sinus; used to designate blood channels in organs such as the heart, liver, spleen, pancreas
- sinusotomy (sinus/otomy)—surgical incision of a sinus
- sinusology (sinus/ology)—that branch of medicine which has to do with the sinuses

---

somato-   body / the body

Examples:

- somal, somatic (som/al, somat/ic)—pertaining to the body
- soma (som/a)—denoting the body as distinguished from the mind

The elements *som-, somat-* are used to refer to the body as a whole, as in:

- somatomegaly (somat/o/megal/y)—abnormal size of a body; giantism
- somatotherapy (somat/o/therap/y)—treatment aimed at curing the ills of the body
- somasthenia (som/asthenia)—a condition of bodily weakness

Or, the elements may be used to emphasize the body as distinct from the mind, as in:
- somatopathy (somat/o/path/y)—a bodily disorder as distinguished from a mental one
- somatopsychic (somat/o/ psych/ic)—pertaining to both body and mind
- psychosomatic (psych/o/somat/ic)—pertaining to the mind-body relationship; having bodily symptoms of a psychic, emotional or mental origin

---

tarso-   ankle region; instep

Examples:
- tarsus (tars/us)—the ankle region
- tarsal (tars/al)—pertaining to the instep; pertaining to the ankle bones (tarsal bones)
- metatarsus (meta/tars/us)—the part of the foot between the ankle (tarsus) and the toes. (Meta- means "beyond," therefore, the literal translation of metatarsus is "beyond the tarsus," "beyond the ankle")
- metatarsal (meta/tars/al)—pertaining to the metatarsus; one of the five bones between the ankle and the toes

---

-top-   place / location

The chief application of this suffix is in the word *isotope* that denotes forms of a chemical element that have identical chemical properties but different atomic weights. So called because they are put in the "same place" in the Periodic Table (classification of elements).

A much wider use is made of the root *top-* meaning "place," "locality," or "local."

-ectopia (-ec/top/ia) is a suffix meaning displacement; literally, "a condition of (ia) out of (ec-) place (top)." The stem is attached to organs or parts indicating such a displacement: oste/o/ec/top/ia, my/ec/top/ia.

The element may have the meaning of "local" or "localized" as opposed to "general" or "widespread:"
- topical (top/ic/al)—pertaining to a particular spot; local; as in topical anesthesia (local anesthesia) versus general anesthesia
- topalgia (top/algia)—fixed or localized pain

 *ectopic- out of place

trachel-   neck or necklike structure

Trachel- applies to a neck or necklike structure and is most frequently used with reference to the neck of the body or the neck (cervix) of the uterus.

Examples:
- trachelocystitis (trachel/o/cyst/itis)—inflammation of the neck of the bladder
- trachelodynia (trachel/odyn/ia)—pain in the neck
- trachelomyitis (trachel/o/my/itis)—inflammation of the muscles of the neck

Another root closely resembling *trachel-* is the element <u>*trache-*</u> that refers to the <u>windpipe</u>, the main trunk of the system of tubes by which air passes to and from the lungs:
- trachea (trache/a)—name of the windpipe
- tracheal (trache/al)—pertaining to the windpipe

Following is a review of the elements denoting a neck or necklike structure that are used interchangeably:
- cervic/o-, trachel/o- —combining forms indicating relationship to a neck or necklike structure
- cervic/itis, trachel/itis—inflammation of the uterine cervic (neck of the womb)

☞   **Note:** trache/itis is inflammation of the trachea (the windpipe)

Lesson 7—Element Recognition

Separate the word terminals, elements, and connecting vowels of the following medical terms from right to left by inserting a slash mark (/) between them.

Example: trachelocystitis—trachel/o/cyst/itis

helio/path/ia
pertaining to a sunlight disease

astr/o/cyt/oma
tumor composed of star shaped cells

lei/asthenia
weak smooth muscles

fasci/o/desis
binding fibrous tissue to tissue attached to the skeleton

iso/genesis

tarso/megal/y
enlarged ankle

top/algia
fixed or localized pain

pod/arthr/itis
inflammation of the foot joints

malignant *tending to become progressively worse, can lead to death if not treated*

adnex/o/genesis
production of appendages

ocul/o/path/y
disease of the eye

lapar/o/chole/cyst/otomy
cutting into the gall bladder & abdominal wall in purpose of RED

dacry/o/cyst/o/rhin/o/stenosis
condition of narrow nose & tear gland

scler/aden/itis
inflammation of hard glands

somat/asthenia
smooth muscles of the body

trachel/o/dyn/ia
pain in the neck

sinus/otomy
cutting into a hollow place for purpose of RED

hypn/o/gen/ic

scirrhoblepharoncus

antr/ostomy
make an opening in a chamber

endo/crin/o/path/y

adnex/ectomy
surgical removal of all or part of the appendages

lapar/o/salping/otomy
cutting into the tubes of the abdomin wall for purpose of RED

dacry/o/aden/algia
pain in the lacrimal gland

scler/o/sten/osis
condition of a ___ ___

somat/esthesia
sensation in the body

trachel/o/my/itis
inflammation of the neck muscle

sinus/itis
inflammation of a hollow place

hypn/algia

antr/ectomy
surgical removal of all or part of a chamber

crin/o/genic

heli/osis
sunstroke

astr/o/cyte

gastr/asthenia
weak stomach

fasci/o/rrhaphy
suturing of torn fibrous tissue

iso/cyt/osis
condition of equal cells

tars/o/pt/osis
condition of ___ angle ___ place

top/esthesia
sensation

pod/o/dyn/ia
pain in the foot

dacry/o/lith/iasis
condition of stones in the tears

somat/o/psychic

sinus/oid
like a hollow place

- 133 -

Lesson 7—Interpretation Exercise

Complete the following statements by printing the meanings of the elements that make up the medical term in the proper blanks. (Remember, most medical terms are interpreted from right to left.)

7-1.   Adnexa is a word that literally means _____ and is applied chiefly to refer to the appendages of the eye and those of the uterus.

7-2.   An antrum (antr/um) is a _____, especially within a bone.

7-3.   The term asthenopia (asthen/op/ia) denotes a condition of _____ in the _____.

7-4.   An astrocytoma (astr/o/cyt/oma) is a _____ consisting of a _____ -shaped _____.

7-5.   Hypercrinia (hyper/crin/ia) refers to _____ _____ of any endocrine gland.

7-6.   Dacryogenic (dacry/o/gen/ic) pertains to the _____ of _____.

7-7.   Dura means _____ and is used as a shortened form of duramater, the outer covering of the brain and spinal cord.

7-8.   The word fascia is used to denote a _____ of fibrous tissue.

7-9.   Heliosensitivity (helio/sensitivity) denotes _____ to the _____.

7-10.   Hypnology (hypn/ology) is the _____ of _____.

7-11.   The term isocellular (iso/cell/ul/ar) refers to the composition of cells of the _____ size or kind.

Lession 6 Test

1 bucco- cheek
2 rug -wrinkle, fold, crease
3 physio- body
4 acoust- hearing
5 stoma- mouth
6 phon- voice
7 phleb- vein
8 plexus- network
9 histo- tissue
10 palpebr- eyelid
11 thalam - switch board of brain
12 ren- kidney
13 cor- heart
14 colpo- hollow /vagina
15 umbilic- navel (belly button)
16 ren/al hypo/plasia - below normal growth of the kidney
17. lei/o/ma - tumor composed of smooth muscle tissue.
18 cili/o/penia - decreased number ~~amount~~ of hairlike projections.
19 crypt/orchid/ism- when testes don't drop

20. hyster/o/salping/ostomy - create an opening between the fallopian tube & uterus.
21 encephal/o/myel/itis- inflammation of the spinal cord & brain

+2
-2
0

good job!

C/B Jamie Neeley

-2 22 de/pil/atory -

23 phlebo/phleb/ostomy - create an opening between
two veins

24 dendr/ite - branch of the nervous system

25 aur/o/salpingo/tympan/o/plast/y - surgical
-2 repair of the ear drum, fallopian tube
of the ear.

what?

x2 E.C. pyo/sal pinx -

7-12. A laparogastrostomy (lapar/o/gastr/ostomy) is the creation of a permanent

_____ to the _____ through the _____ wall.

7-13. The term malignant (malign/ant) is used to denote something _____.

7-14. Dementia (de/ment/ia) is a general term for _____ deterioration.

7-15. The term oculopathy (ocul/o/path/y) refers to any _____of the

_____.

7-16. Prepartal (pre/part/al) denotes occurring just _____ _____.

7-17. The term podalic (pod/al/ic) denotes being accomplished by means of the _____.

7-18. A mastoscirrhus (mast/o/scirrh/us) is a _____ cancer of the _____.

7-19. Sclerosis (scler/osis) is a _____ of _____.

7-20. A septum (sept/um) is general term to designate a dividing _____.

7-21. A sinus is a _____ in the body.

7-22. The term somatopathy (somat/o/path/y) denotes a _____ _____
as distinguished from a mental one.

7-23. Tarsus (tars/us) pertains to the _____ region of the foot.

7-24. The term topalgia (top/algia) denotes _____ _____.

7-25. Trachelomyitis (trachel/o/my/itis) is an _____ of the _____
within the _____.

Lesson 8

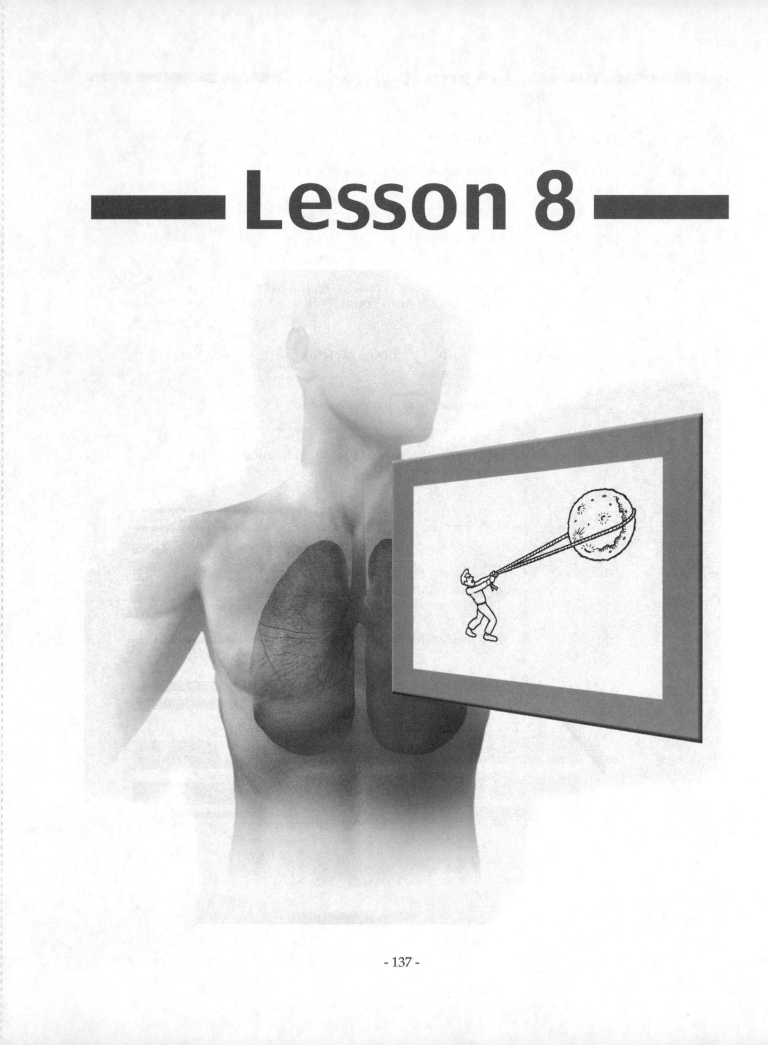

Lesson 8—Review

Element	Audionym	Visual Image	Meaning
pneum-	name (plate)	See the **name** plate turned into a **lung**!	lung
phage	page	See the **page eat**ing!	to eat
phren-	friend	See the boy and girl pulling on the **frien**d saying, **"mine! mine! mine!"**!	mind
corne-	corn	See the **corn** with **horn**s growing out of it!	horny
plak-	plaque	See the **plaque** with a **plate** of food on it!	plate
iris	I race	See the person saying, **"I race"** while racing on a **rainbow**!	rainbow
kerat-	carrot	See the **carrot** with **horn**s growing out of it!	horny
pulmo-	pull moon	See someone **pul**ling on the **moon** that turns into a **lung**!	lung
ptyal-	tile	See the **tile** with a **sail**boat on it!	saliva
alveol-	owl field	See the **owl** in the **field** falling into a **cave-in** (cavity)!	cavity
oophor-	over	See the **over**turned **egg** and **eggs** being turned **over**!	ovary
oment-	O men	See the **"O" men** with a **covering** over their heads!	covering

Element	Audionym	Visual Image	Meaning
sedat-	seated	See the speaker saying, "Be **seated**" and the audience becoming **quiet** and **calm**!	quiet, calm
furca-	fur coat	See the **fur coat** covered with **fork**s!	fork-shaped
radic-	radish	See the **radi**sh with the **root** beer bursting out of it!	root
radi-	radio	See the **radi**o with a **ray** of light beaming out of it!	ray
fistul-	fist	See the **fist** full of **pipe**s!	pipe
edema	a demon	See **a dem**on **swelling** and **swelling**!	swelling
dactyl-	duck tail	See the **duck tail** with a **finger** and **toe** growing out of it!	finger, toe
metabol(e)	met a bull	See the man who **met a bul**l asking it for **change**!	change
pariet-	parrot	See the **parrot** with **walls** on its sides!	wall
ependym-	a pendulum	See **a pendu**lum with **wrapping** all over it!	wrapping
gravid	gravel	See the sacks of **grav**el with **pregnant** women sitting on them!	pregnant
aer-	airplane	See the **air**plane with **air** coming out of it in all directions!	air
glyco-	glide coal	See the **gli**ding **co**al made of **sweet** chocolate!	sweet

Lesson 8—Worksheet

Print the audionym and meaning of the elements in the proper blanks:

Element	Audionyn	Meaning
pneum-		
phage		
phren-		
corne-		
plak-		
iris		
kerat-		
pulmon-		
pulmo-		
ptyal-		
alveol-		
oophor-		
oment-		
sedat-		
furca-		
radic-		
radi-		
fistul-		
edema		
dactyl-		
metabol(e)		
pariet-		
ependym-		
gravid		
aer-		
glyco-, gluco-		

Lesson 8—Review

Element	Audionym	Visual Image	Meaning
sedat-	seated	See the speaker saying, "Be **seated**" and the audience becoming **quiet** and **calm**!	quiet, calm
furca-	fur coat	See the **fur coat** covered with **fork**s!	fork-shaped
radic-	radish	See the **radi**sh with the **root** beer bursting out of it!	root
radi-	radio	See the **radi**o with a **ray** of light beaming out of it!	ray
fistul-	fist	See the **fist** full of **pipe**s!	pipe
edema	a demon	See **a dem**on **swelling** and **swelling**!	swelling
dactyl-	duck tail	See the **duck tail** with a **finger** and **toe** growing out of it!	finger, toe
metabol(e)	met a bull	See the man who **met a bull** asking it for **change**!	change
pariet-	parrot	See the **parrot** with **walls** on its sides!	wall
ependym-	a pendulum	See **a pendu**lum with **wrapping** all over it!	wrapping
gravid	gravity	See the image for **gravi**ty, a **pra**ying nut falling from a tree!	pregnant
aer-	airplane	See the **air**plane with **air** coming out of it in all directions!	air
glyco-	glide coal	See the **gli**ding **co**al made of **sweet** chocolate!	sweet

Print the audionym and meaning of the elements in the proper blanks:

Element	Audionyn	Meaning
pneum-	_____	_____
phage	_____	_____
phren-	_____	_____
corne-	_____	_____
plak-	_____	_____
iris	_____	_____
kerat-	_____	_____
pulmon-	_____	_____
pulmo-	_____	_____
ptyal-	_____	_____
alveol-	_____	_____
oophor-	_____	_____
oment-	_____	_____
sedat-	_____	_____
furca-	_____	_____
radic-	_____	_____
radi-	_____	_____
fistul-	_____	_____
edema	_____	_____
dactyl-	_____	_____
metabol(e)	_____	_____
pariet-	_____	_____
ependym-	_____	_____
gravid	_____	_____
aer-	_____	_____
glyco-, gluco-	_____	_____

Lesson 8—Word Terminals

-ization	action or process

This terminal is a combination of *-ize* and *-ation*.

-ize to do, to act in a specified way

Examples:
- liquid/ize, union/ize, critic/ize, brutal/ize

-ation (see Word Terminals, Lesson 4) a process, action or condition

Examples:
- commercial/ization, real/ization, crystall/ization

-ity	condition; character

Examples:
- formal/ity, normal/ity, civil/ity

-ive	of, relating to, having the nature or quality of

Examples:
- nat/ive, substant/ive, sedat/ive, direct/ive

-or	a person or thing that does something or has some particular function

In Lesson 3 the terminal *-or* was defined as "that which does something or has some particular function." All we are doing here is including "a person or thing" as one of the "that which does."

Examples:
- invent/or, object/or, elevat/or, sail/or, vend/or

-ence	is another form of *-ance* (Word Terminals, Lesson 7) and means the same thing, that is, "a state or condition; the act of"

aer-   air / gas

This element represents an older spelling of air and persists in medical terminology. It is used to indicate air or an otherwise unspecified gas.

Examples:

- aerial (aer/i/al)—pertaining to the air
- aerosis (aer/osis)—the production of gas in the tissues or organs of the body
- aeropathy (aer/o/path/y)—any disease due to a change in atmospheric pressure such as compressed air illness ("bends") or air sickness

alveol-   cavity; socket / small cavity, pit or hollow

This root is used most frequently in reference to the cavities or sockets of either jaw in which the roots of the teeth are embedded. (Note: Cavity as used here is a hollow space and does not refer to the pits in the teeth resulting from decay which are more properly dental caries.)

Examples:

- alveolus (alveol/us)—(plural alveoli) name used to designate a small saclike pit or cavity
- dental alveoli (dent/al alveol/i)—the tooth sockets in the upper and lower jaw bones
- alveolar (alveol/ar)—pertaining to an alveolus
- alveolectomy (alveol/ectomy)—surgical excision of the tooth socket bony structure as a preparatory measure for the wearing of false teeth (dent/ures); may include the removal of remaining teeth and roots of teeth and excision of diseased tissue
- alveoloplasty (alveol/o/plast/y)—the surgical improvement of the shape and condition of the tooth sockets in preparation for immediate or future denture construction

corne-   horny, hornlike / the cornea of the eye, the transparent part of the covering of the eyeball that covers the iris and pupil and admits light to the interior _callus_

[handwritten margin note: clear covering of the eye]

Examples:

- corn—the name of a build-up of thick horny skin tissue produced by friction and pressure
- corneal (corne/al)—pertaining to the cornea of the eye
- corneous (corne/ous)—hornlike or horny

dactyl-   finger; toe / digit (Note: a digit is a finger or a toe; a finger is a "digit of the hand," a toe is a "digit of the foot.")

Examples:

- dactyloscopy (dactyl/o/scop/y)—examination of fingerprints for purpose of identification

    ☞ **Note:** In medical terminology the fingers and toes are technically called digits; although the element *dactyl-* applies to fingers and toes, it is more frequently used for the fingers.

Examples:

- isodactylism (iso/dactyl/ism)—a condition in which the fingers are of relatively equal length
- dactylospasm (dactyl/o/spasm)—a spasm or cramp of a finger or toe

-dactylia, sometimes -dactyly (-dactyl/ia, -dactyl/y)—a condition of the fingers or toes

edema   swelling by fluid / an abnormal accumulation of fluid in cells, tissues or cavities of the body, resulting in swelling

Edema is a word that can be used to form terms such as "edema of _____" or as a prefix (meaning "pertaining to") or as a suffix (referring to location or fluid accumulation).

Examples:

- edematous (edemat/ous)—pertaining to or affected by edema
- pneumonedema (pneumon/edema)—abnormal quantities of fluid in the lungs
- dactyledema (dactyl/edema)—abnormal swelling of the fingers or toes due to fluid accumulation

ependym-   wrapping; a covering / specifically, the membrane lining the cavities of the brain and the canal enclosing the spinal cord

Examples:

- ependyma (ependym/a)—name of the membrane lining the cavities of the brain and the canal enclosing the spinal cord
- ependymal (ependym/al)—pertaining to or composed of ependyma
- ependymopathy (ependym/o/path/y)—any disease of this membrane (the ependyma)
- ependymitis (ependym/itis)—inflammation of the ependyma

fistul-   ~~pipe~~ *channel*; a narrow passage / an abnormal passage leading from an abscess (a collection of pus in a cavity) or hollow organ to the body surface, or from one hollow organ to another and permitting passage of fluids (as pus) or secretions (as saliva)

Examples:
- fistula (fistul/a)—term for such an abnormal passage
- fistulous (fistul/ous)—pertaining to or of the nature of a fistula

Fistulas are described by their location:
internal fistula—an abnormal passage between two internal organs
external fistula—an abnormal passage between a hollow organ and the external surface of the body
intestinal fistula—an abnormal passage connecting with the intestine

Sometimes a fistula may be surgically created as a therapeutic measure:
- fistulization (fistul/ization)—the process of becoming fistulous; the surgical creation of an opening into a hollow organ or of an opening between two structures which were not previously connected
- fistuloenterostomy (fistul/o/enter/ostomy)—the operation of making a fistula empty permanently into the intestine

furca-   fork-shaped / frequently used to designate the area between the roots of the teeth

Examples:
- furcal (furc/al)—shaped like a fork; forked
- bifurcate (bi/furc/ate)—forked; divided into two like a fork (*bi-* means "two" and is discussed more fully in Lesson 12)
- bifurcation (bi/furc/ation)— division into two branches; the site where a single structure divides into two

glyco-, gluco-   sweet; sugary / sugar

This root is chiefly used to indicate the presence of sugar in the blood:
- glycemia (glyc/em/ia)—the presence of sugar in the blood
- hyperglycemia (hyper/glyc/ em/ia)—abnormally increased content of sugar in the blood

Examples:
- glycolysis (glyc/o/lysis)—the breaking down of sugar into simpler compounds
- glycopenia (glyc/o/penia)—a deficiency of sugar in the body tissues
- glucose (gluc/ose)—a thick, syrupy, sweet liquid; the sweet, colorless, soluble form of dextrose that occurs widely in nature and is the usual form in which carbohydrate is assimilated by animals

gravid pregnant

Examples:
- gravid—pregnant; containing developing young
- gravidic (gravid/ic)— occurring during pregnancy
- gravidity (gravid/ity)—the condition of being with child; pregnancy
- gravidocardiac (gravid/o/cardi/ac)—pertaining to heart disease of pregnancy

iris rainbow (eye membrane) / specifically, the colored membrane of the eye

Examples:
- iris—name of the colored membrane of the eye
- iridic, sometimes iridal (irid/ic, irid/al)— pertaining to the iris
- iridization (irid/iz/ation)—the patient's perception of colored halos about lights, occurring in glaucoma (a disease of the eye marked by increased pressure within the eyeball)

cornea - callus

kerat- horny; horny tissue / also the cornea of the eye

Examples:
- keratic (kerat/ic)—pertaining to horny tissue; pertaining to the cornea
- keratoderma (kerat/o/derma)—a horny skin or covering
- keratoid (kerat/oid)—resembling horny or corneal tissue
- hyperkeratosis (hyper/kerat/osis)—overgrowth (excessive growth) of the horny layer of the skin
- keratomalacia (kerat/o/malacia)—softening of the cornea
- keratocentesis (kerat/o/ centesis)—puncture of the cornea

Comparison between kerat/o- and corne-:

kerat/o- is used to designate horny tissues and relationship to the cornea

corne- is used principally to designate the cornea of the eye as a structure and landmark

metabol(e) change

Examples:
- metabolism (metabol/ism)—the sum of all the physical and chemical processes by which living organized substance is produced and maintained, and also the transformation by which energy is made available for the use of the body
- basal metabolism—the minimal energy needed to maintain the physical and chemical activities of the body

oment- covering (of internal abdominal organs) / the membrane in the front part of the abdomen that folds over and supports the stomach, liver and parts of the intestine

apron

Examples:
- omentum (oment/um)—name of the membranous cover of the abdominal organs
- omental (oment/al)—pertaining to the omentum
- omentopexy (oment/o/pexy)—the attachment of the omentum to another tissue or organ
- omentoplasty (oment/o/plast/y)—the use of omental grafts, that is, surgical repair using the omentum as the grafting material

oophor- ovary / literally "egg carrier" (oo-, egg or ovum + phor-, carrier); either of the pair of female reproductive glands producing eggs and sex hormones

As is indicated above the elements *oophor-* and *ovar-* are synonyms, *ovar-* being more frequently used to designate the anatomical part and *oophor-* being more frequently used to name diseases, abnormalities and therapeutic procedures applied to these reproductive glands.

Examples:
- oophoron (oophor/on)—an ovary
- oophoropexy (oophor/o/pexy)—the surgical fixation or attaching of the ovary (also called adnexopexy [adnex/o/pexy]; you will recall that an adnexus is an appendage or attachment. The ovaries [oophor-] the uterine tubes [salping-], and the ligaments are considered as appendages of the uterus [uterine adnexa].)
- hystero-oophorectomy (hyster/o/oophor/ectomy)— surgical removal (excision) of the uterus and ovaries (also called oophor/o/hyster/ectomy)

pariet- wall / wall of an organ or cavity

This element may be used to denote a wall or a side of an organ or cavity of the body. It is used chiefly to designate two bones that form the side walls of the cranium, the parietal bones.

Example:
- parietal (pariet/al)—pertaining to the walls of a cavity
- parietitis (pariet/itis)—inflammation of the wall of an organ

phage to eat / eating, swallowing

Examples:
- onychophagy (onych/o/phag/y)—nail biting
- phagomania (phag/o/mani/a)—an insatiable craving for food; literally an "eating mania"

- phagocyte (phag/o/cyt/e)—any cell that absorbs ("eats") micro-organisms, other cells, and foreign bodies
- phagocytosis (phag/o/cyt/osis)—the process of engulfing a micro-organism, other cells and foreign bodies by phagocytes
- odynophagia (odyn/o/phag/ia)—pain in swallowing

phren-   mind / also the ~~diaphragm~~; also the phrenic nerve, a nerve with branches spreading mostly over the lower part of the diaphragm

The diaphragm is the muscular wall or partition separating the chest cavity and the abdominal cavity; the "midriff."

Examples:
- phrenic (phren/ic)—pertaining to the mind; pertaining to the diaphragm
- phrenic- (phren/ic-)—form denoting relationship to the phrenic nerve

The suffix *-phrenia* is used to form words having to do with mental disorders:

- bradyphrenia (brady/phren/ia)—slowness of mental activity such as initiative, interest, speech, frequently accompanying encephalitis

☞   **Note:** The ancient Greeks, from whose language this root is taken, believed that the diaphragm was the location of the mind just as we, today, believe that the head (actually the brain) is the location of the mind. It would have been as commonplace for the Greeks to describe a person as having a good "diaphragm" as for us to describe a person as having a good "head"; both usages would indicate a good "mind."

crud

plak-   ~~a plate~~ / also plaque; a patch of eruption

This root appears in the form -plak/ia and indicates a forming of patches of eruption, usually on mucous membrane:
- leukoplakia (leuk/o/plak/ia)—a disease marked by white thickened patches on the mucous membrane of the cheeks, gum and tongue
- malacoplakia (malac/o/plak/ia)—the formation of soft patches on the mucous membrane of a hollow organ

plaque—any patch or flat area

dental plaque—a deposit of material on the surface of a tooth

pneum-   the lungs; air

pneum-, pneumat- forms indicating a relationship to air or to respiration (the inhalation and exhalation of air):
- pneumal (pneum/al)—pertaining to the lungs

lungs or air

- pneumatic (pneumat/ic)—of or pertaining to air or respiration
- pneumatocele (pneumat/o/cele)—a swelling containing air any place in the body; a pushing out of the lung through a weak place in the wall of the chest

pneumon- form indicating a relationship to the lungs

- pneumonia (pneumon/ia)—inflammation of the lungs, usually with complications and usually accompanied by chill, increase in temperature, pain and coughing
- pneumonitis (pneumon/itis)—a condition of localized, acute inflammation of the lung without the range of complications and symptoms accompanying pneumonia; benign pneumonia
- pneumonic (pneumon/ic)—pertaining to the lung or to pneumonia

The importance of air to maintain life is reflected in the various forms in which the element *pne-* is applied in the formation of medical terms. The presence of the root *pne-* in a word indicates a relationship to air or breathing.

-pnea (-pne/a)—breathing

- hyperpnea (hyper/pne/a)—abnormal increase in the speed and depth of breathing
- hypopnea (hypo/pne/a)—abnormal decrease in the speed and depth of breathing
- bradypnea (brady/pne/a)—abnormal slowness of breathing

---

ptyal- saliva / spit

Examples:
- ptyalism (ptyal/ism)—excessive secretion of saliva; salivation
- *-ptysis (-pty/sis)—the spitting of
  - hemoptysis (hem/o/pty/sis)—the spitting of blood or of blood stained spittle (sputum)
- ptyalectasis (ptyal/ectasis)—dilatation (enlarging) of a salivary duct by surgery
- ptyalogenic (ptyal/o/gen/ic)—formed from or by the action of saliva

---

pulmon- lung

Examples:
- pulmo (pulm/o)—the lung, the organ of respiration
- pulmonic, pulmonary (pulmon/ic, pulmon/ary)—pertaining to the lungs

-pulmonary (-pulmon/ary) is used as a suffix denoting relationship to the lungs and the preceding element:
- renopulmonary (ren/o/pulmon/ary)—pertaining to the kidney and lungs

hemoptysis-spitting blood

Comparison of *pulm/o, pulmon/o-* with *pneumon/o:*

pulm/o- and pulmon/o- are used, principally, to indicate the lung as a landmark

pneumon/o- is used principally to name conditions and therapeutic procedures applied to the lungs

---

radi- ray; beam; spoke

This root is used to convey the idea of something that spreads out from the center like spokes from the hub of a wheel; it is used particularly in medicine to denote the process whereby energy in the form of light, heat and X-rays is emitted.

Examples:
- radial (radi/al)—pertaining to rays; pertaining to the spreading out from the center
- radiology (radi/ology)—the study of X-rays, frequently called roentgenology after Wilhelm Konrad Roentgen, the discoverer of X-rays
- radiotherapy (radi/o/therap/y)—the treatment of disease by the use of X-rays or rays from a radioactive substance

---

radic- root / origin

Examples:
- radical (radic/al)—directed to the cause; going to the root or source of a morbid process
- radix—"the root"; the lowermost part, or a structure by which something is firmly attached
- radicle (radi/cle)—"a little root"; any one of the smallest branches of a vessel or nerve

The form *radicul-* (radic/ul-) usually denotes a nerve root, particularly the spinal nerve roots:
- radiculectomy (radic/ul/ectomy)—excision of a nerve root
- radiculoneuropathy (radic/ul/o/neur/o/path/y)—disease of the nerve roots and the nerve (*neur-* is a root meaning "nerve" and is discussed more fully in Lesson 10)

---

sedat- quiet; calm

Examples:
- sedation (sedat/ion)—the act or process of calming
- sedative (sedat/ive)—an agent such as a drug that calms or reduces excitement

Lesson 8—Element Recognition

Separate the word terminals, elements, and connecting vowels of the following medical terms from right to left by inserting a slash mark (/) between them.

Example: oophorocystectomy—oophor/o/cyst/ectomy

pneum/o/melan/osis
condition of black lung

phag/o/cyt/o/lysis
destruction of cells that eat microorganisms

phren/asthenia
weak diaphragm

irid/ectasis
expansion of the eye membrane

kerat/o/gen/esis
production of callus

pulmon/itis
inflammation of the lungs

ptyal/o/lith/iasis
condition of stones in the saliva

alveol/o/dont/al
pertaining to a cavity in the tooth

oophor/o/hyster/ectomy
surgical removal of all or part of the ovaries of the uterus

oment/o/rrhaphy
suturing of the covering of the internal organs

sedat/ive
to make quiet or calm

furc/al
being fork-shaped

radi/ectomy
surgical removal of the root of a tooth

radi/o/carcin/o/gen/esis
production of cancer due to rays

fistul/ectomy
surgical removal of all or part of a narrow passage

cephal/edema
fluid swelling in the head

dactyl/o/spasm
involuntary contractions of the fingers or toes

metab/o/logy
the study of change

pariet/itis
inflammation of the wall of an organ

ependym/itis
inflammation of the membrane enclosing the brain & spinal cord

gravid/o/cardi/ac
pertaining to the heart disease during pregnancy

aer/enter/ectasia
expansion of the small intestine due to gas

hyper/glyco/derm/ia
more than normal sugar in the skin

alveol/algia
pain in the socket

oment/itis
inflammation of the covering of the internal organs

radic/al
pertaining to the root

dactyl/o/gram
finger print

metabol/ism
an abnormal condition of change

ependym/o/cyte
a cell membrane enclosing the brain & spinal cord

aer/end/o/cardi/a
disease of air within the heart

glyc/o/penia
decrease of sugar

pneum/o/hypo/derm/a
under the skin amount of skin on the lungs

phag/o/mania
an insatiable craving for food

phren/itis
inflammation of the diaphragm

irid/o/ptosis
drooping of the colored part of the eye

kerat/o/derma
callus on the skin

pulmon/ectomy
surgical removal of all or part of the lung

ptyal/o/genic
production of saliva

phren/o/pathy
disease of the diaphragm

kerat/oma
tumor composed of hard tissue

ptyal/o/lith/otomy
to cut into saliva stones

ependym/a
the membrane enclosing the brain & spinal cord

Lesson 8 — Interpretation Exercise

Complete the following statements by printing the meanings of the elements that make up the medical term in the proper blanks. (Remember, most medical terms are interpreted from right to left.)

8-1.   The term aerial (aer/i/al) denotes pertaining to the _____.

8-2.   Alveolus (alveol/us) is the name used to designate a small saclike _____.

8-3.   Corneous (corne/ous) refers to being _____.

8-4.   Dactyloscopy (dactyl/o/scop/y) is the _____ of _____-prints for the purpose of identification.

8-5.   Dactyledema (dactyl/edema) is an abnormal _____ of the _____ or _____ due to fluid accumulation.

8-6.   The ependyma (ependym/a) is the name of the _____ that lines the cavities of the brain and the canal enclosing the spinal cord.

8-7.   A fistula (fistul/a) is a term for an abnormal _____ leading from an abscess or hollow organ.

8-8.   The term furcal (furc/al) denotes being shaped like a _____.

8-9.   Hyperglycemia (hyper/glyc/em/ia) refers to an abnormal _____ of _____ in the blood.

8-10.   The word gravid means _____.

8-11.   The iris is the _____ membrane of the eye.

8-12.   Hyperkeratosis (hyper/kerat/osis) is a condition of over-growth of the _____ layer of skin.

8-13.   Metabolism (metabol/ism) is the _____ by which energy is made available for use by the body.

8-14.   The omentum (oment/um) is the _____ in the front part of the abdomen which folds over and supports the stomach, liver and parts of the intestines.

8-15.   Oophoron (oophor/on) is another name for an _____.

8-16.   The term parietal (pariet/al) pertains to the _____ of a cavity.

8-17.   Odynophagia (odyn/o/phag/ia) denotes _____ when _____.

8-18.   Bradyphrenia (brady/phren/ia) denotes a _____ of _____ activity.

8-19.   Leukoplakia (leuk/o/plak/ia) is a disease marked by _____ thickened _____ or patches.

8-20.   Pneumonitis (pneumon/itis) is an _____ of the _____.

8-21.   The term ptyalogenic (ptyal/o/gen/ic) pertains to being formed from or by the action of _____.

8-22.   The term renopulmonary (reno/pulmon/ary) denotes pertaining to the _____ and _____.

8-23.   Radiotherapy (radi/o/therap/y) is the treatment of disease by use of _____ from a radioactive source.

8-24.   The radix is the _____ part of a structure by which something is firmly attached.

8-25.   A sedative (sedat/ive) is an agent such as a drug that _____.

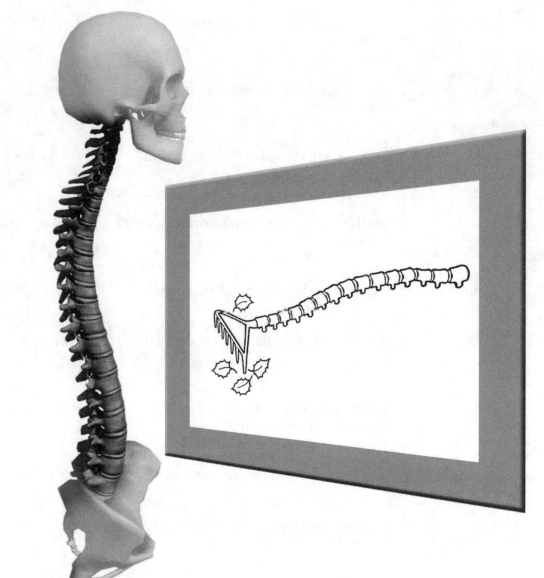

Lesson 9 — Review

Element	Audionym	Visual Image	Meaning
tarso-	tar	See the **tar** with the **framework of the eyelid** in it!	framework of the eyelid
cheir-	care (care package)	See the **Care** Package with a **hand** sticking out of it!	hand
calc-	calculator	See the **calc**ulator with a **heel** and a **stone** on it!	heel, stone
cine-	Sen Sens	See the **Sen Sens** (mints) **moving** on their own!	move
digit	dig it (shovel)	See the image of **"dig it"** (shovel) with a **finger** and **toe** on it!	finger, toe
dors-	doors	See the double **doors** with a **back** on each of them!	back
gangli-	gang	See the **gang swelling** and **swelling**!	swelling
gemin-	gem	See the **gem**s that are **twins** and exactly alike!	twin
grad-	graduate	See the **grad**uate **walk**ing away and **taking** the **steps** with her!	walk, take steps
gran-	grandma	See **gran**dma eating **grain particles**!	grain, particle
labi-	lab (test tube)	See the image for **lab**, a test tube with **lip**s on it!	lip
micr-	microphone	See the **micr**ophone that is very, very **small**!	small

Lesson 9 — Review

Element	Audionym	Visual Image	Meaning
peps-	Pepsi	See the **Peps**i bottle with the Readers **Digest** stuck into it!	digest
pleur-	pliers	See the **pleur**s with **rib**s on its **side**s!	pleura, rib, side
mamm-	mammal (whale)	See the **mamm**al (whale) made of a **breast!**	breast
colla-	cola	See the **cola** filled with **glue**!	glue
later-	ladder	See the **ladder** with someone climbing up the **side** of it!	side
rachi-	rake	See the **rake** made of a **spinal column**!	spinal column
phob-	foe	See the **foe** with a shield made of **fur**!	fear
phot-	photo	See the **phot**o with a **light** shining out of it!	light
dys-	dice	See the **dice** with a **bat** stuck through them!	bad
cut-	cut (scissors)	See the "**cut**," (scissors) made of **skin**!	skin
en-	hen	See the h**en** saying, "they won't let me **in** the **in**n"!	in
peri-	pear	See the **pear** having **a bout** with **a round** pear!	about, around
pro-	pro	See the **pro** golfer with people walking **in front of** the ball **before** the pro can hit it!	in front of, before

Print the audionym and meaning of the elements in the proper blanks:

Element	Audonym	Meaning
tarso-		
cheir-, chir-		
calc-		
cine-		
digit		
dors-		
gangli-		
gemin-		
grad-		
gran-		
labi-		
micr-		
peps-, pept-		
pleur-		
mamm-		
colla-		
later-		
rachi-		
phob-		
phot-		
dys-		
cut-		
en-		
peri-		
pro-		

Lesson 9 — Reading Assignment

calc-	heel; stone / basically refers to calcium, one of the essential materials in the body

This element may appear as *calc-* referring to the element calcium:
- calcic (calc/ic)—of, or pertaining to, calcium
- calcemia (calc/em/ia)—the presence of an abnormally large amount of calcium in the blood

Or, it may appear as *calcan-* referring to the heel bone:
- calcaneus (calcane/us)—name of the heel bone, the large tarsal (ankle) bone that forms the heel

Or, it may appear as *calcare-* referring to the various chemical compounds containing calcium; lime and chalky substances are chemical forms containing calcium:
- calcareous (calcare/ ous)—pertaining to or containing lime or calcium; chalky

cheir-, chir-	hand

Examples:
- chiropractic (chir/o/pract/ic)—a method of treating disease by manipulation of the body, especially manipulation of the spine with the hands
- chiropractor (chir/o/pract/or)—one who practices chiropractic
- cheirarthritis (cheir/arthr/itis)—inflammation of the joints of the hands including the joints of the fingers

cine-	move; movement / also kine-

The form *cine-* is used principally to refer to the use of photographic or motion picture techniques in studying motion in the various organs such as the heart.

Examples:
- cineradiography (cine/radi/o/graph/y)— the making of motion picture records of images produced by X-rays
- cineangiography (cine/angi/o/graph/y)—the recording of images of the blood vessels through motion picture techniques
- cineangiocardiography (cine/angi/o/cardi/o/graph/y)—the recording of images of the heart and blood vessels through motion picture techniques

The form *kine-* is used to denote the more general relationship to movement:

- kine-, kinesi- (kine/si-)—forms denoting relationship to movement
- kinemia (kin/em/ ia)—movement of the blood from the heart
- kinesitherapy (kines/i/therap/y)—the treatment of disease by movements or exercise

-kinesia, -kinesis (-kines/ia, -kine/ sis)—combinations meaning abnormal movement:

- bradykinesia (brady/kines/ia)—slow movement

Another form, *kinet-*, is used with the meaning "movable":

- kinet- form meaning "movable"
- kinetic (kinet/ic)—pertaining to or producing motion
- kinetism (kinet/ism)—the ability to perform or begin muscular motion

colla-   glue; gelatinlike; starch

Examples:
- collagen (colla/gen)—the gelatinlike or sticky substance of skin, bone, cartilage and connective tissue
- collagenous (colla/gen/ous)—forming or producing collagen; pertaining to collagen
- collagenogenic (colla/gen/o/gen/ic)—pertaining to the production of collagen
- colloid (coll/oid)—gelatinlike or resembling glue or starch

cut-   skin

Examples:
- cutis (cut/is)—the skin; the outer protective covering of the body
- cuticle (cut/icle)—"a little skin"; the outer layer of the skin; the ep/onych/ium
- cutitis (cut/itis)—inflammation of the skin

Cutaneous (cutan/ eous) is a word meaning skin. It is used frequently as a suffix denoting relationship to the skin:
- subcutaneous (sub/cutan/eous)—situated or occurring beneath the skin
- transcutaneous (trans/cutan/eous)—through the skin

digit   finger; toe / medical word used to name a finger or a toe

Example:
- digital (digit/al)—pertaining to the digits (fingers or toes) (See discussion of dactyl—Lesson 8)

dors-   back / the back of the body; the body as viewed from the back

This root is used principally to denote the back of the body or the back of any body part as a landmark; the meaning would be close to "back side."

Examples:

- dorsum (dors/um)—name for the back; the back of the body
- dorsal (dors/al)—pertaining to the back or the "back side"; denoting a position more toward the back surface than to some other object of reference
- dorsad (dors/ad)—toward the back or the "back side"
- subdorsal (sub/dors/al)—situated below the dorsal (back) region
- dorsolateral (dors/o/later/al)—pertaining to the back and side

dys-   bad; out of order / difficult; painful; opposite of "good"

Examples:

- dysentery (dys/enter/y)—abdominal disorders marked by inflammation of the intestines and accompanied by pain in the abdomen, cramp and frequent bowel movements containing blood and mucus
- dyspepsia (dys/peps/ia)—indigestion; a weakening or lessening of the power or function of digestion
- dysphagia (dys/phag/ia)—difficulty in swallowing
- dyspnea (dys/pne/a)—difficult or labored breathing
- dystrophy (dys/trophy)—a disorder arising from defective or faulty nutrition; faulty development

en-   in / within; inside; usually em- before b, m, or p

Examples:

- encephal- (en/cephal-)—"within the head"; usually with reference to the brain; however, the reference may be to other conditions within the head as, for example, encephalalgia, "pain within the head" or headache
- enostosis (en/ost/osis)—an abnormal bony growth developed within the cavity of a bone
- empathy (em/path/y)—"feeling within"; the entering into the feelings of another person
- emplastic (em/plast/ic)—literally "pertaining to forming within"; adhesive; a constipating medicine

gangli-   swelling; knotlike mass

This root denotes relationship to a ganglion: ganglion (gangli/on)—a normal mass of nerve cells outside of the brain and spinal column; or, an abnormal tumor or cyst consisting of tendon tissue and usually appearing on a wrist or an ankle.

Examples:
- gangliocytoma (gangli/o/cyt/oma)—a tumor containing ganglion cells
- ganglioplexus (gangli/o/plex/us)—a network (plexus) of nerve fibers in a ganglion
- ganglionectomy (gangli/on/ectomy)—excision of a ganglion

gemin-   twin, double / paired

Examples:
- geminate (gemin/ate)—paired; occurring in pairs; also called bi/gemin/al
- geminus (gemin/us)—a twin
- gemini (gemin/i)—twins

grad-   walk; take steps / a stage in a process

Graduated (grad/u/ated) means marked by a progression of lines, steps or degrees:
- graduate (grad/u/ate)—a container marked with a series of lines used to measure volume / one who receives a degree.

-grade (-grad/e)—suffix indicating a series of steps; a progression:
- retrograde (retr/o/grad/e)—going backward
- digitigrade (digit/i/grade)—characterized by walking on the toes

gran-   grain, particle

Examples:
- granul- (gran/ul-)—form denoting relationship to small particles
- granule (gran/ul/e)—a small particle
- granulation (gran/ul/ation)—the formation in wounds of small rounded fleshy masses
- granuloma (gran/ul/oma)—a tumor composed of grainy tissue
- granuloplastic (gran/ul/o/plast/ic)—forming granules

labi-   lip / any liplike structure, especially the lips of the face

The root *labi- is* the landmark reference for a lip or liplike structure; the root *cheil-* is used to designate conditions of or therapy applied to the lip.

Examples:

- labium (labi/um)—a fleshy border or edge; used as a general term to designate such a structure
- labial (labi/al)—pertaining to a lip; pertaining to a labium
- labiodental (labi/o/dent/al)—pertaining to the lips and teeth
- labiology (labi/ology)—the study of the movements of the lips in singing and speaking

later- side / the side of the body

Examples:

- lateral (later/al)—pertaining to a side; also, denoting a position farther from the middle or the midline of the body or of a structure
- laterad (later/ad)—toward a side
- lateroposition (later/o/position)—displacement to one side
- laterality (later/al/ity)—a tendency to use the organs (hand, foot, ear, eye) of the same side

mamm- breast

Examples:

- mammi-, mammo- (mamm/i-, mamm/o-)—forms denoting relationship to the breast or the milk secreting gland in the breast of the female (the mast/aden-)
- mamma (mamm/a)—name for the breast
- mammary (mamm/ary)—pertaining to the breast
- mamill- —an element used to denote the nipple of the breast or any nipplelike structure (note the dropping of the double "m" [mam(m)] and the use of a double "l" at the end; the literal meaning of this element is "little breast")
- mamilla (mamill/a)—name for the nipple or any nipplelike structure
- mammoplasty (mamm/o/plasty)—plastic reconstruction of the breast
- mammogram (mamm/o/gram)—x-ray of the breast

The root *mast- is* used to designate the female breast and the mammary gland (the milk secreting gland) and the diseases and corrective procedures relating to the female breast and mammary gland:

- mastalgia (mast/algia)—pain in the mammary gland
- mastectomy (mast/ectomy)—excision of the breast; mammectomy

micr- small / small size; minute, that is, "microscopic"

This root is widely used in medical terms to convey the idea of "smallness." Micr /_____ ia or micr /_____ y—forms used to designate abnormally small body structures, such as:

- microblepharia (micr/o/blephar/ia)—small eyelids
- microcephaly (micr/o/cephal/y)—small head
- microcardia (micr/o/card/ia)—small heart

The root may be used to distinguish smaller from larger structures, such as:

- microaden- (micr/o/aden-)—small glands, usually small lymph glands
- microangi- (micr/o/angi-)—small blood vessels
- microscope (micr/o/scop/e)—an instrument used to obtain a large image of small objects
- microscopic (micr/o/scop/ic)—of extremely small size; visible only by the aid of a microscope
- microsurgery (micr/o/surgery)—dissection of small structures under the microscope

The root can serve to illustrate some of the distinctions in the use of synonymous or related elements:

- microphthalmia (micr/ophthalm/ia)—abnormal smallness of the eyes
- micropsia (micr/ops/ia)—a condition in which objects are seen as smaller than they usually are
- micrencephaly (micr/en/cephal/y)—abnormal smallness of the brain
- micropsychia (micr/o/psych/ia)—literally "a condition of small mind"; feebleness of the mind, feeble-minded

peps, pept-   digest / digestion

Examples:

- pepsin (peps/in)—a substance secreted in the stomach that begins the digestive process
- peptic (pept/ic)—pertaining to digestion, such as a peptic ulcer (an ulcer is an open sore; other than a wound on the skin or some mucous membrane) which is an ulcer on the lining of the stomach; pertaining to pepsin

-pepsia (-peps/ia)—word termination denoting a condition of digestion:

- dyspepsia (dys/peps/ia)—faulty digestion; indigestion
- bradypepsia (brady/peps/ia)—slow digestion

peri-   about, around / surrounding; enclosing; covering

This prefix is used widely in medical terms to designate the area or space around a body part (the "vicinity" or "neighborhood"); the tissue that encloses and frequently supports or lubricates a part.

In the sense of the area or space around a part:

- periodontal (peri/odont/al)—situated or occurring around a tooth
- periosteoma (peri/oste/oma)—a morbid bony growth surrounding a bone
- periadenitis (peri/aden/itis)—inflammation of the tissues around a gland

In the sense of a tissue that covers, surrounds, or encloses a part, peri/o/_____/ium, peri/o/_____/eum are forms used to name the enclosing or covering tissue of a part:

- periosteum (peri/oste/um)—a specialized connective tissue covering all bones of the body
- pericardium (peri/card/ium)—the fibrous sac that surrounds the heart

---

phob-   fear / persistent abnormal fear or dread

Examples:

- phobia (phob/ia)—a condition or state of abnormal fear
- phobe, -phobe (phob/e, -phob/e)—one having a specified phobia
- phobic, -phobic (phob/ic, -phob/ic)—of the nature of or pertaining to phobia or morbid fear

-phobia (phob/ia)—word termination designating abnormal fear of or aversion to the subject indicated by the preceding element to which it is affixed:

- phobophobia (phob/o/phob/ia)—a condition marked by fear of one's own fear

---

phot-   light

Examples:

- photic (phot/ic)—pertaining to light
- photoallergy (phot/o/allergy)—an allergic type of sensitivity to light
- photophobia (phot/o/phob/ia)—abnormal intolerance of light
- photosensitive (phot/o/sensitive)—sensitive to light
- photo-ophthalmia (phot/o/-ophthalm/ia)—blindness or severe inflammation of the eye caused by intense light such as an electric light, rays of welding arc, or reflection from snow

---

pleur-   pleura (membrane)
          rib, side

Examples:

- pleura (pleur/a)—name for the membrane that covers the lungs and lines the thoracic (chest) cavity
- pleural (pleur/al)—pertaining to the pleura
- pleurisy, pleuritis, (pleur/isy, pleur/itis)—inflammation of the pleura
- pleuropneumonia (pleur/o/pneumon/ ia)—pleurisy complicated with pneumonia
- pleurocholecystitis (pleur/o/chole/cyst/itis)—inflammation of the pleura and the gallbladder

pro-   in front of; before / front part of

> Examples:
> - prolabium (pro/labi/um)—the prominent central part of the upper lip
> - prolapse (pro/lapse)—a slipping forward (or out of place) of an organ or part of the body; a displacement (lapse means "a fall")
> - proptosis (pro/ptosis)—a forward displacement
> - prootic (pro/ot/ic)—situated in front of the ear
> - proencephalon (pro/en/cephal/on)—the front part of the brain

rachi-   spinal column / spine; the backbone; the vertebral column

> Examples:
> - rachis (rachi/s)—name for the spinal column
> - rachidial, rachidian (rachidi/al, rachidi/an)—pertaining to the spinal column
> - rachitis (rach/itis)—inflammation of the spine; a disease commonly known as rickets, in which there is a failure to form bones properly and a softening of the bones because of a lack of vitamin D
> - rachitic (rach/it/ic)— pertaining to or affected with rickets or rachitis
> - rachicentesis (rachi/centesis)—puncture into the spine

tarso-   framework of the eyelid

> We learned tarso- in Lesson 7 with the meaning "ankle." The element is re-introduced in order that you may remember another meaning, "framework of the eyelid."
>
> Examples:
> - tarsus of the lower eyelid (tars/us)—the edge of the lower eyelid
> - tarsus of the upper eyelid (tars/us)—the edge of the upper eyelid
> - tarsitis (tars/itis)—inflamation of the tarsus or edge of the eyelid; blepharitis

Lesson 9—Element Recognition

Separate the word terminals, elements, and connecting vowels of the following medical terms from right to left by inserting a slash mark (/) between them.

Example: dorsocephalad—dors/o/cephal/ad

tarsocheiloplasty

cheiropodalgia

calculogenesis

cineplasty

dorsalgia

graduated

granulocytopenia

labiomycosis

microangiopathy

peptogenic

mammoplasia

lateral

rachiodynia

phagophobia

photodermatosis

dysosteogenesis

subcutaneous

encephalomeningopathy

mammoplasty

periglossitis

proptosis

pleuralgia

mammectomy

rachiotomy

topophobia

photesthesis

dyscholia

cutitis

encephalalgia

pericerebral

proglossis

tarsitis

cheirarthritis

calcaneodynia

cinesalgia

granulocyte

labiology

microlithiasis

pleurocholecystitis

dysendocrinia

encysted

periosteoma

Lesson 9—Interpretation Exercise

Complete the following statements by printing the meanings of the elements that make up the medical term in the proper blanks. (Remember, most medical terms are interpreted from right to left.)

9-1.   A calculus (calc/ul/us) is a small _____ as found in the gall bladder, kidney or urinary bladder.

9-2.   Cheirarthritis (cheir/arthr/itis) is an _____ of the _____ of the _____ including those of the fingers.

9-3.   Cineradiography (cine/radi/o/graph/y) refers to the graphic presentation of images produced by x-rays through _____ picture techniques.

9-4.   The term collagenous (colla/gen/ous) denotes the formation of collagen the _____ -like substance.

9-5.   The term cutis (cut/is) pertains to the _____.

9-6.   Digit is the medical word for a _____ or _____.

9-7.   The term dorsolateral (dors/o/later/al) pertains to the_____ and _____.

9-8.   The term dysphagia (dys/phag/ia) denotes _____ _____.

9-9.   Encephalalgia (en/cephal/algia) denotes pain _____ the _____.

9-10.   The term ganglion (gangli/on) is used to denote a _____ of nerve cells and tendon tissue.

9-11.   To geminate (gemin/ate) is to arrange or form in _____.

9-12. The term digitigrade (digit/i/grad/e) denotes _____ on the _____.

9-13. A granule (gran/ul/e) is a small_____.

9-14. The term labiodental (labi/o/dent/al) pertains to the _____ and the _____.

9-15. Lateral (later/al) denotes pertaining to a _____.

9-16. A mammogram (mamm/o/gram) is the _____ of an x-ray of the _____.

9-17. The term microcardia (micr/o/card/ia) refers to a _____ _____.

9-18. The term bradypepsia (brady/peps/ia) denotes _____ _____.

9-19. Periadenitis (peri/aden/itis) is an _____ of the tissue _____ a _____.

9-20. A phobia (phob/ia) is a term denoting abnormal _____.

9-21. Photosensitive (phot/o/sensitive) denotes sensitivity to _____.

9-22. The pleura (pleur/a) is the name of the _____ that covers the lungs and lines the thoracic cavity.

9-23. The term proencephalon (pro/en/cephal/on) pertains to the_____ of the _____.

9-24. Rachicentesis (rachi/centesis) denotes the _____ of the _____ _____.

9-25. Tarsitis (tars/itis) is an inflammation of the _____ of the eyelid.

Lesson 10

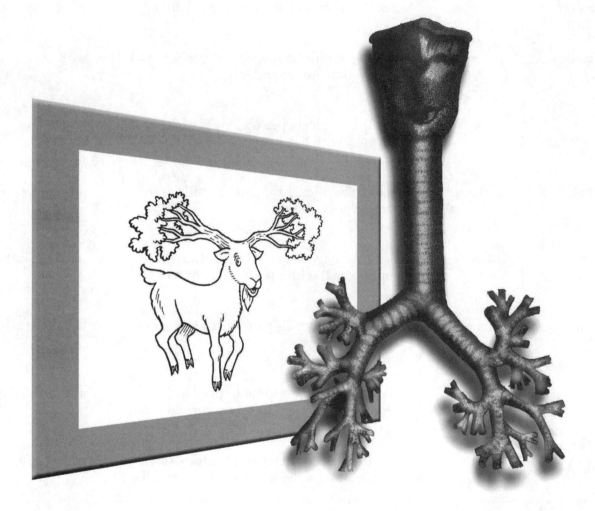

Element	Audionym	Visual Image	Meaning
mechano-	mechanic	See the **mechan**ic with a washing **machine** strapped on his back!	machine
dynam-	dynamite	See the **dynam**ite exploding with **power** saws bursting out of it!	power
osmo-	I smoke	See the man saying **I smo**ke **"O" do**ors!	odor
traumat-	laundromat	See the laun**dromat** with the washers and dryers that are **wound**ed!	wound
trich-	trick	See the magician performing a **trick** covered with **hair**!	hair
maxill-	makes hill	See the bulldozer that **makes hil**ls with an **upper jawbone**!	upper jawbone
an-, a-	an "A"	See the image of **an "A"** (the student's report card) **without** an "A", **not** one "A"!	without, not
phak-	vacuum (cleaner)	See the **vacuum** cleaner with a huge **lens** on it!	lens
pre-	pray	See the people stopping to **pray in front of** the church **before** entering!	in front of, before
strict-	strict	See the **strict** parent using a rope **draw**n **tight**ly around the teenagers to control them!	draw tight
turbin-	turban	See the **turban shaped like a top**!	shaped like a top
ameb-	a me	See the person looking into the mirror asking "**a me**" for **change**!	change

Element	Audionym	Visual Image	Meaning
semi-	semi (semi-colon)	See the **semi**-colon cut in **half**!	half
neo-	kneel	See the people **kneel**ing on a **new** carpet!	new
hormone	harmonize	See the couple **harmon**izing with everyone heading to the **exit**!	excite
therm-	thermometer	See the **therm**ometer producing **heat**!	heat
syn-, sym-	cymbals	See the **cym**bals stuck **together**!	together
vuls-	false (false teeth)	See the **false** teeth with **two witch**es **pull**ing them!	twitch or pull
post	post (post office)	See the **post** office with someone arriving **after** it closed!	after
metr-	meter	See the **meter** pointers saying, "You turn us"!	uterus
tegument	tag you men	See the image for "**tag** you **men**," the men playing tag **cover**ed with **skin**!	covering, skin
pan-	pan	See the **pan** containing **all** the food in the house!	all
poly-	polish	See the shoe **poli**sh made of **many** colors!	many
ramus	ram	See the **ram** with **branch**es instead of horns!	branch
neuro-	Nero	See **Nero** being very **nervous** as Rome burns!	nerve (nervous system)

Lesson 10—Worksheet

Print the audionym and meaning of the elements in the proper blanks:

Element	Audionym	Meaning
mechano-	_____	_____
dynam-	_____	_____
osmo-	_____	_____
traumat-	_____	_____
trich-	_____	_____
maxill-	_____	_____
an-, a-	_____	_____
phak-	_____	_____
pre-	_____	_____
strict-	_____	_____
turbin-	_____	_____
ameb-	_____	_____
semi-	_____	_____
neo-	_____	_____
hormone	_____	_____
therm-	_____	_____
syn- or sym-	_____	_____
vuls-	_____	_____
post	_____	_____
metr-	_____	_____
tegument	_____	_____
pan-	_____	_____
poly-	_____	_____
ramus	_____	_____
neuro-	_____	_____

Lesson 10—Reading Assignment

ameb-   change / a parasite that moves by changing shape

Examples:
- ameba, amoeba (ameb/a, amoeb/a)—a one-celled animal that moves by constantly changing its shape; amebas (amoebas) are found in soil and water and some varieties exist as parasites in human tissues and cavities
- amebic (ameb/ic)—pertaining to, or of the nature of, an ameba
- amebiasis (ameb/ia/sis)—infestation with amebas, especially with a variety that is a parasite in the intestines

an-, a-   without, not / lacking; weakness; deficiency

This is a widely used prefix that can be attached to words to indicate the negative or opposite aspect of the word to which it is prefixed. Most of the applications in medical terms carry the meaning of "without" in the sense of "lacking," "being deficient in," "weakness in."

☞   **Note:** The form of the prefix is *an-* before vowels (a, e, i, o, u) and usually h; the form is *a-* before all other letters (the consonants).

Examples:
- anemia (an/em/ia)—"lack of blood"; lack of red cells in the blood
- anesthesia (an/esthesia)— "lack of feeling"; unconsciousness
- avitaminosis (a/vitamin/osis)—"lack of vitamins"; a disease caused by vitamin deficiency
- atrophy (a/trophy)— "lacking development, growth"; a wasting away or a decrease in the size of a cell, tissue, organ or part due to a defect of nutrition

dynam-   power / force; strength

Examples:
- dynamic (dynam/ic)—pertaining to or exhibiting force
- adynamia (a/dynam/ia)—lack or loss of normal powers; asthenia
- myodynamic (my/o/dynam/ic)—relating to muscular force
- hyperdynamia (hyper/dynam/ia)—excessive muscle activity
- cardiodynamics (cardi/o/dynam/ics)—science of the motions and forces involved in the heart's action

hormone   to excite or set in motion / applied to a substance formed in an organ of the body (principally the glands) and carried by a body fluid to another organ or tissue where it has a specific effect such as stimulation or arousal

Examples:
- hormonic (hormon/ic)—pertaining to or acting as a hormone; having the exciting influence of a hormone
- hormonotherapy (hormon/o/therap/y)—treatment by the use of hormones
- hyperhormonal (hyper/hormon/al)—pertaining to hormone excess
- hypohormonal (hypo/hormon/ al)—pertaining to hormone deficiency

---

maxill-   upper jawbone

Examples:
- maxilla (maxill/a)—name of the upper jawbone. There are two such bones, the left maxilla and the right maxilla, that are joined at the center of the face.
- maxillary (maxill/ary)— pertaining to the maxilla
- maxillectomy (maxill/ectomy)—surgical removal of the maxilla
- maxillolabial (maxill/o/labi/al)—pertaining to the upper jawbone and the lip

---

mechano-   machine

Examples:
- mechanotherapy (mechano/therap/y)—the use of mechanical apparatus (machines) in the treatment of disease; especially as an aid in performing therapeutic exercises
- mechanism (mechan/ism)—this word, formed from the root mechan-, is used in medical terminology to designate a system or a mental or physical process by which some result is produced:
  - labor mechanism (mechanism of labor)—the process involved in the expulsion of the infant and the afterbirth through the birth canal in labor
  - defense mechanism—any self-protective physiological reaction of an organism; in psychiatry, any behavior or thought process unconsciously brought into use by an individual to protect himself against painful or anxiety-provoking feelings and impulses

---

metr-   uterus / womb / hyster-; female organ for protection and nourishment of the developing young during pregnancy

metr- is used interchangeably with *hyster-* (Lesson Two) to refer to the uterus. The tendency is to use *hyster-* as the root to denote surgical procedures i.e. hysterectomy (hyster/ectomy) the surgical removal of the uterus. The root *metr-* is most used to denote structural parts and conditions:
- metrectasia (metr/ectas/ia)—dilation of the uterus (non-pregnant)
- metritis (metr/itis)—inflammation of the uterus
- metralgia (metr/algia)—pain in the uterus
- metrectopia (metr/ec/top/ia)—displacement of the uterus
- endometritis (endo/metr/itis)—inflammation of the mucus membrane lining of the uterus

When used as a word ending, *-metra (-metr/a)* denotes a condition of the uterus. We are accustomed to *-ia* as a word terminal denoting condition; the *-a* terminal with *metr-* is an exception:

- hematometra (hemat/o/metr/a)—an accumulation of blood in the uterus

---

neo- new / recent

Examples:

- neonatal (neo/natal)—"new born"; pertaining to the first four weeks after birth
- neopathy (neo/path/y)—a new disease; a new condition or complication of disease in a patient
- neoplasm (neo/plasm)—any new and abnormal growth such as a tumor

In Lesson 1 we learned *plast-* and in Lesson 6, *-plasia*. Both of these elements contain the root *plas-* that denotes the idea of forming or formation. The suffix *-plas/m* indicates formative or formed material. In medical terms the reference is usually to the formation of cells or tissues.

---

neuro- nerve or nervous system

Examples:

- neuron (neur/on)—a nerve cell
- neural (neur/al)—pertaining to a nerve or the nerves
- psychoneurosis, neurosis (psych/o/neur/osis, neur/osis)—both terms are used to designate any of various psychic or mental disturbances, characterized by one or several of such reactions as: anxiety, compulsions and obsessions, phobias, depression, etc.

-neuria (-neur/ia)—suffix denoting a condition of nerve function:

- dysneuria (dys/neur/ia)—impairment of the nerve function
- gastrohyperneuria (gastr/o/hyper/ neur/ia)—excessive activity of the nerves of the stomach

-neurium (-neur/ium)—suffix denoting a nerve tissue:

- perineurium (peri/neur/ium)—the connective tissue cover around the nerve fibers

---

osmo- odor / smell; the sense of smell

Examples:

- osmics (osm/ics)—the science that deals with the sense of smell; the study of odors
- osmatic, -osmatic (osmat/ic, -osmat/ic)—pertaining to the sense of smell
- osmophobia (osmo/phob/ia)—irrational fear of odors
- anosmatic (an/osmat/ic)—having no sense of or only an imperfect sense of smell

  -osmia (-osm/ia)—suffix denoting a condition of the sense of smell:
  - anosmia (an/osm/ia)—absence of the sense of smell
  - hyposmia (hyp/osm/ia)—abnormally decreased sensitiveness to odor

pan-   all / completely; the whole of (also pant-)

> Examples:
> - panhysterectomy (pan/hyster/ectomy)—the removal by surgery of the whole of the uterus
> - pancarditis (pan/card/itis)—inflammation of all of the heart, that is, the outer covering (peri/card/itis), the muscular wall (my/o/card/itis) and the lining of the cavities of the heart (end/o/card/itis)
> - pantosomatous (pant/o/somat/ous)—pertaining or relating to the whole body
> - pantalgia (pant/algia)—pain over the whole body

phak-   lens / the crystalline lens of the eye, that is, the transparent body of tissue behind the pupil of the eye that focuses the incoming light rays

> Examples:
> - phakitis, also phacitis (phak/itis, phac/itis)—inflammation of the crystalline lens of the eye
> - phacocele (phac/o/cele)—the displacement of the eye lens from its proper place; hernia of the eye lens
> - phacocyst- (phac/o/cyst-)—form denoting relationship to the sac enclosing the crystalline lens of the eye

poly-   many or much / sometimes with the idea of excessive

> Examples:
> - polyacoustic (poly/acoust/ic)—"much sound"; increasing or intensifying sound
> - polycythemia (poly/cyt/hem/ia)—excessive number of red corpuscles in the blood
> - polyemia (poly/em/ia)—excessive amount of blood in the body
>
> The prefix may be used to indicate a condition involving many of a kind of body part or organ:
> - polyadenitis (poly/aden/itis)—inflammation of several or many glands; similarly poly/aden/oma, poly/aden/o/path/y, poly/aden/osis
> - polydysplasia (poly/dys/plas/ia)—faulty development in several types of tissue or several organs or systems of organs

post   after, behind in time / also, situated behind (behind in place)

> Examples:
> - postpneumonia (post/pneumon/ia)—following pneumonia
> - postoral (post/or/al)—situated behind the mouth
> - postnatal (post/natal)—after the occurrence of birth

The prefix *poster-* is a form denoting relationship to the rear part or back part:
- posterior (poster/ior)—situated in the back part of, or affecting the back part of an organ
- posteriad (poster/i/ad)—toward the posterior part of the body
- posterolateral (poster/o/later/ al)—situated behind and to one side

pre-   in front of; before / situated before, or in front of; occurring before, or prior to, or earlier than

Examples:
- prerenal (pre/ren/al)—situated in front of the kidney
- prepartal (pre/part/al)—occurring before, or just previous, to labor
- prenatal (pre/nat/al)—existing or occurring before birth
- preoperative (pre/operative)—preceding an operation
- precranial (pre/crani/al)—in the front part of the cranium

ramus   branch / a branch or branchlike projecting part

There are many networks in the body that can be described as branching, for example, the nervous system, the circulatory system (arteries, veins and capillaries). These may be called branches or, with the addition of complex Latin terms, be called ramus. In lesson 6 we learned *dendr-* meaning "branch." *Dendr-* is used almost exclusively to indicate the branch of a nerve cell. All other branches are designated as ramus.

Examples:
- ramitis (ram/itis)—inflammation of a root(s)
- ramose (ram/ose)—branching; having many branches

semi-   half / one-half; partially

Examples:
- semilunar (semi/lunar)—resembling a crescent or halfmoon
- semimalignant (semi/malign/ant)—somewhat (partially) malignant
- seminormal (semi/normal)—one-half the normal

strict-   to draw tight; narrowing

Examples:
- stricture (strict/ure)—the abnormal narrowing of a canal, duct or passage
- spastic stricture (spast/ic strict/ure)—a stricture due to a muscle spasm
- stricturotomy (strict/ur/otomy)—the cutting of a stricture

syn- or sym-   together

Examples:

- syndesis (syn/desis)—a "binding together"; the fusion of a joint; arthrodesis
- syndactyly (syn/dactyl/y)—"finger (digit) togetherness"; the most common congenital defect, affecting the hand in which adjacent digits are more or less attached to each other by a membranous web
- symphysis (sym/phy/sis)—a "natural togetherness"; a type of joint in which the connected bones are firmly united such as the joint formed by the various bone parts in the hip
- synalgia (syn/algia)—"pain together"; pain experienced in one place as the result of a soreness or injury in another place

tegument   skin or covering

The word tegument is a shortened form for integument which generally means "a covering" but is widely used to denote the skin.

Examples:

- integumentary (integument/ary)—pertaining to or composed of skin; serving as a covering, like the skin
- the integumentary system (sometimes called common integument)—a term used to designate the entire covering of the body including, not only the skin, but the other body coverings: hair, nails and the skin glands, including the breast, or mammary gland

therm- heat

Examples:

- thermal, thermic (therm/al, therm/ic)—pertaining to or characterized by heat

-thermia, -thermy (-therm/ia, -therm/y)—suffixes donating a state of heat; the generation of heat:

- diathermy (dia/therm/y)—the generation of heat in the body tissues for medical or surgical purposes, usually by the application of electrical currents (*dia-* is a prefix meaning "through" so that, literally, diathermy means "the act of heating through")
- hyperthermia (hyper/therm/ia)—an abnormally high body temperature; fever

traumat-   wound; injury / shock; stress

This element is used to denote relationship to a wound or injury (a trauma).

Examples:

- traumatology (traumat/ology)—the study and treatment of wounds and injuries
- traumatogenic (traumat/o/genic)—produced or caused due to a wound or injury

- traumatic (traumat/ic)—pertaining to, occurring as the result of, or causing trauma

Trauma (traum/a) is:

1. a bodily injury or wound caused by the application of external force or violence such as sprains, bruises, fractures, dislocations, concussions, burns, etc.

2. a psychological or emotional stress or blow that may produce disordered feelings or behavior

- psychic trauma (psych/ic traum/a)—an emotional shock that makes a lasting impression on the mind, especially the subconscious mind

trich- hair

Examples:

- trichoesthesia (trich/o/esthesia)—"hair feeling"; the sense by which one perceives that the hair of the skin is being touched
- trichogenous (trich/o/gen/ous)—promoting the growth of hair

-trichia, -trichosis (-trich/ia, -trich/osis)—conditions of the hair:
- leukotrichia (leuk/o/trich/ia)—whiteness of the hair
- sclerotrichia (scler/o/trich/ia)—hard, dry state of the hair
- atrichosis (a/trich/osis)—absence of the hair; baldness

turbin- shaped like a top / spiral-shaped

Used principally in medical terms with reference to a turbinate, which is one of several spiral spongy bony projections in the nasal passages (the nostrils).

Examples:

- turbinal (turbin/al)—shaped like a top; one of the turbinates
- turbinotomy (turbin/otomy)—the surgical cutting of a turbinate
- turbinectomy (turbin/ectomy)—the surgical removal of a turbinate bone

vuls- twitch or pull / pluck; tear loose

This element is most familiar in convulse and convulsion applied to the violent, irregular motion of a limb or other part of the body due to involuntary contraction of the muscle (the prefix *con-* means "together"; the literal translation of *convuls-* is "a pulling together").

The root also appears in avulsion (sometimes evulsion) that describes the forcible tearing or pulling out of a part in surgery (the prefix *a-* is a form of *ab-* meaning "from" or "away from" that will be discussed more fully in Lesson 11; the literal translation of *avuls-* is "pulling away from"):

- nerve avulsion (a/vuls/ion)—the operation of pulling a nerve from its origin
- avulsion, nail plate (a/vuls/ion)—the pulling out of a diseased or infected outer layer of the nail of a finger or toe

Lesson 10—Element Recognition

Separate the word terminals, elements, and connecting vowels of the following medical terms from right to left by inserting a slash mark (/) between them.

Example: trichorrhexis—trich/o/rrhexis

dynamogenesis

osmesthesia

traumatopathy

trichotrophy

maxillectomy

anesthesia

phacosclerosis

pretympanic

stricturotomy

turbinectomy

ameboid

neophrenia

hormonogenesis

thermohyperesthesia

syndactylism

postcardiotomy

metrophlebitis

panhematopenia

polytrichia

neurotrophasthenia

turbinotomy

ameba

neophobia

thermalgesia

synchilia

metrocolpocele

pancytolysis

polypathia

neurootology

dynamoscopy

osmophobia

traumatologist

trichorrhexis

maxillitis

analgesia

phacomalacia

precostal

thermolysis

synosteology

metrostenosis

polycheiria

neurotrauma

Complete the following statements by printing the meanings of the elements that make up the medical term in the proper blanks. (Remember, most medical terms are interpreted from right to left.)

10-1.　An ameba (ameb/a) is a one celled animal that moves by ＿＿＿＿＿＿ its shape.

10-2.　The term anemia (an/em/ia) denotes the ＿＿＿＿＿＿ of ＿＿＿＿＿＿.

10-3.　The term myodynamic (myo/dynam/ic) relates to＿＿＿＿＿＿ ＿＿＿＿＿＿.

10-4.　Hypohormonal (hypo/hormon/al) pertains to a hormone ＿＿＿＿＿＿.

10-5.　The maxilla (maxill/a) is the name of the ＿＿＿＿＿＿ ＿＿＿＿＿＿.

10-6.　Mechanotherapy (mechano/therap/y) denotes the use of ＿＿＿＿＿＿ in the treatment of disease especially in performing therapeutic exercise.

10-7.　Hematometra (hemat/o/metr/a) refers to an accumulation of ＿＿＿＿＿＿ in the ＿＿＿＿＿＿.

10-8.　The term neopathy (neo/path/y) denotes a ＿＿＿＿＿＿ ＿＿＿＿＿＿.

10-9.　Neural (neur/al) pertains to a ＿＿＿＿＿＿.

10-10. Osmics (osm/ics) refers to the science dealing with ＿＿＿＿＿＿.

10-11. A panhysterectomy (pan/hyster/ectomy) is the surgical ＿＿＿＿＿＿ of the ＿＿＿＿＿＿ ＿＿＿＿＿＿.

10-12. Phakitis (phak/itis) is an ＿＿＿＿＿＿ of the ＿＿＿＿＿＿ of the eye.

10-13 The term polyacoustic (poly/acoust/ic) denotes _____ _____.

10-14. Postoral (post/or/al) refers to situated _____ the _____.

10-15. The term precranial (pre/crani/al) denotes being situated in the _____ of

the _____.

10-16. A ramus is a _____ -like projection.

10-17. The term semimalignant (semi/malign/ant) denotes being _____

_____.

10-18. A stricture (strict/ure) is abnormal _____ of a canal; duct; passage.

10-19. The term syndesis (syn/desis) denotes _____.

10-20. Tegument is a word meaning "a _____" and is widely used to denote

_____.

10-21. Hyperthermia (hyper/therm/ia) denotes_____ _____.

10-22. A trauma (traum/a) is a bodily _____ caused by an external force
or violence.

10-23. The term leukotrichia (leuk/o/trich/ia) denotes _____ of
the _____.

10-24. The term turbinal (turbin/al) denotes being shaped like a _____.

10-25. A convulsion (con/vuls/ion) is the violent irregular motion of the body due to the
involuntary _____ of the muscles.

Lesson 11

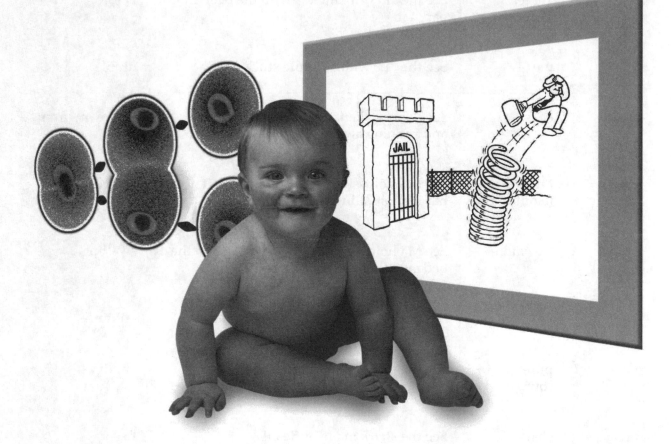

Element	Audionym	Visual Image	Meaning
thromb-	trombone	See the **tromb**one with a **lump** or a **clot** stuck in it!	lump, clot
ab-	Abe (Lincoln)	See **Ab**e sneaking **away from** the Capitol to tie k**not**s!	away from, not
-plegia	pledge	See the people **pledg**ing allegiance and becoming **paralyzed**!	paralysis
ante-	ant tea	See the **ant** drinking **tea** with the **beef** and **oar** in it!	before
thel-	the "L"	See **the "L"** with a **nipple** stuck on it!	nipple
ex-	eggs	See the **eggs** jumping **out** of the carton and running **away**!	out, away from
lien-	line (clothesline)	See the clothes**line** with students on it having a **spelling** bee!	spleen
tumor	two more	See Ma holding **two more** children and the bed **swelling** and **swelling**!	swelling
vestibule	vest bull	See the **vest** on the **bull** that's an **entrance**!	entrance
puer-	pure (pure gold)	See the **pure** gold **child**!	child
sarc-	shark	See the **shark** made of **flesh**!	flesh
proli-	parolee	See the **parolee** jumping **off** the **spring**!	offspring
macro-	macaroni	See the **mac**aroni that is very very **large**!	large

Element	Audionym	Visual Image	Meaning
lal-	lollipop	See the **lol**lipop presenting a **speech**!	speech
intra-	introduce	See the woman being **intro**duced to someone **within** the man!	within
inter-	interpreter	See the **inter**preter. She is a **bee** in **tweed**!	between
infra-	infrared (infrared oven)	See the **infra**red oven with a **bee** on its **knee**s inside it!	beneath
cryo-	cry	See the baby **cry**ing because it is **cold** sitting on an igloo!	cold
mal-	mall	See the **mal**l with baseball **bat**s shopping!	bad
glom-	glow	See the **glo**w in the sky with **ball**s falling out of it!	ball
tens-	tents	See the **tents stretch**ed!	stretch
spas-	space	See the **space** vehicle **pulling** another vehicle with someone **drawing** in it!	pull, draw
somni-	"saw my knee"	See the woman saying, "He **saw my knee**" because I was **sleep**ing!	sleep
pharmac-	farm axe	See the **"farm axe"** made of a **drug**store!	drug
lumbo-	lumber	See the **lumb**er with **lions** coming out of it!	loins

Print the audionym and meaning of the elements in the proper blanks:

Element	Audionym	Meaning
thromb-	_____	_____
ab-	_____	_____
-plegia	_____	_____
ante-	_____	_____
thel-	_____	_____
ex-	_____	_____
lien-	_____	_____
tumor	_____	_____
vestibule	_____	_____
puer-	_____	_____
sarc-	_____	_____
proli-	_____	_____
macro-	_____	_____
lal-	_____	_____
intra-	_____	_____
inter-	_____	_____
infra-	_____	_____
cryo-	_____	_____
mal-	_____	_____
glom-	_____	_____
tens-	_____	_____
spas-	_____	_____
somni-	_____	_____
pharmac-	_____	_____
lumbo-	_____	_____

Lesson 11—Reading Assignment

ab- away from

This prefix takes the form *a*- before m, p and v and *abs*-before c and t.

Examples:
- abnormal (ab/normal)—away from normal; departing from normal
- abneural (ab/neur/al)— passing from a nerve (usually to a muscle)
- avulsion (a/vuls/ion)—"a pulling away from"; This word was discussed in Lesson 10 under vulse but is introduced here to help in understanding the "away from" meaning of *a*- as a form of *ab*-.

ante- before / before in time (occurring before); before in space (situated in front of or at the front of)

Examples:
- antepartum (ante/part/um)—occurring before birth
- antelocation (ante/ location)—the forward (toward the front) displacement of an organ

This prefix appears in a frequently used form *anter/o*- which is restricted to the meaning "before in space (situated in front)" or "forward" and usually carrying the idea of direction:

- anterior (anter/ior)—situated more toward the forward part of an organ; used freely to designate the belly surface of the body
- anteroposterior (anter/o/poster/ior)—from front to back

cryo- cold

Examples:
- cryotherapy (cryo/therap/y)—the therapeutic use of cold
- cryosurgery (cryo/surgery)—the destruction of tissue by extreme cold as, for example, the treatment of malignant tumors of the skin
- cryoextraction (cryo/extraction)—the application of low temperature in the removal of a body part such as a cataract
- hematocryal (hemat/o/cry/al)— cold blooded

ex- out; away from / out of; outside of

Examples:
- exostosis (ex/ost/osis)—a condition (bony growth) projecting outward from the surface of a bone

- extensor (ex/tens/or)—that which stretches (extends) as, for example, a muscle which extends a joint

The element *ex-* may appear in several forms.

exo- meaning "outside"; "outward"; "outer":
- exogenic (exo/gen/ic)—"produced outside"; developed or originating outside the body
- exopathy (exo/path/y)—"disease outside"; a disease originating in some cause lying outside the body

extra- meaning "outside of"; "beyond":
- extracardial (extra/cardi/al)—outside the heart
- extrahepatic (extra/hepat/ic)—situated or occurring outside the liver

ecto- situated on the outside; outside:
- ectosteal (ect/oste/al)—pertaining to or situated on the outside of a bone
- ectocytic (ecto/cyt/ic)—outside the cell

---

glom- ball / a rounded mass; a cluster; in the form of a ball; a tuft

This root is used chiefly in medical terminology to denote two kinds of small anatomical structures:
- glomus (glom/us)—a small round anatomical (normal) swelling made up of tiny blood vessels
- glomic (glom/ic)—pertaining to a glomus
- glomerulus (glomer/ul/us)—a tufted structure or a cluster generally composed of blood vessels or nerve fibers; used principally to designate coils of blood vessels in the kidney
- glomerul- (glomer/ul-)—form for a glomerulus
- glomerular (glomer/ul/ar)—pertaining to or of the nature of a glomerulus

---

infra- beneath / situated or occurring below or beneath

Examples:
- inframammary (infra/mamm/ary)—situated below the mammary gland
- inframaxillary (infra/maxill/ary)—beneath the jaw
- infracostal (infra/cost/al)—beneath the ribs or beneath a rib
- infrapsychic (infra/psych/ic)—below the psychic (mind) level; non-thinking; automatic

---

inter- between / situated, formed or occurring between

This prefix is used widely to designate a location between or among the parts or structures named in the second element to which it is affixed.

Examples:
- interlabial (inter/labi/al)—between lips
- interosseous (inter/oss/eous)—between bones
- intermuscular (inter/muscul/ar)—between muscles
- interdigital (inter/digit/al)—between adjacent fingers or toes

intra- within / situated within

This prefix is used widely with the meanings "situated within" or "occurring within."

Examples:
- intraspinal (intra/spin/al)—situated or occurring within the vertebral column
- intraoperative (intra/operative)—performed or occurring within the course of a surgical operation

A variation of intra- is the prefix *intro-* carrying the meaning "into"; frequently "insertion into."

lal- speech / babbling

Examples:
- lalopathy (lal/o/path/y)—any disorder of speech
- lalophobia (lal/o/phob/ia)—fear or extreme dislike of speaking (stage fright), often associated with stuttering

-lalia (-lal/ia)—a speech disorder:
- echolalia (echo/lal/ia)—the meaningless repitition by a patient of words addressed to him
- rhinolalia (rhin/o/lal/ia)—a nasal quality of voice due to some disorder or defect of the nasal passages
- bradylalia (brady/lal/ia)—abnormally slow speech due to a brain disorder

lien- spleen / the fist-sized organ near the stomach in the upper part of the abdomen that modifies and stores blood

Examples:
- lienal (lien/al)—pertaining to the spleen
- lien—name for the spleen
- gastrolienal (gastr/o/lien/al)—pertaining to the stomach and the spleen
- lienorenal (lien/o/ren/al)—pertaining to the spleen and the kidney

lumbo- loins / the sides of the back lying on each side of the spinal column between the end of the ribs and the hipbone

Examples:
- lumbar (lumb/ar)—pertaining to the loins

- lumbago, lumbodynia (lumb/ago, lumb/odyn/ia)— pain in the lumbar region; "lower back pains"
- dorsolumbar (dors/o/lumb/ar)—pertaining to the back and loins
- supralumbar (supra/lumb/ar)—situated above the loins
- sublumbar (sub/lumb/ar)— situated below the loins

---

macro-   large / enlargement

This root carries the meaning large or of abnormal size or length. The form for abnormal size or length is usually macr/_____/ia or macr/_____/y.

Examples:
- macropsia (macr/ops/ia)—"large vision"; a disturbance of vision in which objects are seen as larger than they really are
- macrophthalmia (macr/ophthalm/ia)—"large eyes"; abnormal enlargement of the eyeballs
- macrostomia (macro/stom/ia)—"big mouth"; greatly exaggerated width of the mouth
- macrotooth (macro/tooth)—an abnormally large tooth
- macrodontia (macr/odont/ia)— abnormal increase in the size of the teeth

---

mal-   bad / irregular; abnormal; faulty; poor (in the sense of inadequate or insufficient)

Examples:
- maldigestion (mal/digestion)—faulty or impaired digestion
- malformation (mal/formation)—defective or abnormal formation; deformity
- malpractice (mal/practice)—improper or injurious practice; unskillful and faulty medical or surgical treatment

Remember *malign-* taught in Lesson 7. It also means bad but most always with the association of getting progressively worse.

---

pharmac-   drug / medicinal drug; medicine

Examples:
- pharmacy (pharmac/y)—the art of preparing, compounding and dispensing medicines; a drug store (in the sense of a store or shop in which prescription drugs are prepared and dispensed)
- pharmacal (pharmac/al)—pertaining to pharmacy
- pharmacopsychosis (pharmac/o/psych/osis)—a term for any one of the group of mental diseases due to alcohol, drugs or poison
- photopharmacology (phot/o/pharmac/ology)—the study of the effects of light and other radiations on drugs

-plegia   paralysis / a stroke; a loss of power

Examples:
- panplegia (pan/plegia)—(also pam/plegia) total paralysis
- hemiplegia (hemi/plegia)—paralysis of one side of the body

proli-   offspring / production

Examples:
- prolific (proli/fic)—fruitful; productive (-*fic* is an ending meaning "causing," "bringing about")
- proliferous (proli/fer/ous)—characterized by the production of offspring (-*ferous* is an ending meaning "bearing," "producing")

puer-   child / children

Examples:
- puerile (puer/ile)—pertaining to childhood or to children; childish
- puerper- (puer/per-)—combination denoting relationship to childbirth
- puerpera (puer/per/a)—a woman who has just given birth to a child; a new mother
- puerperium (puer/per/ium)—the period or state of confinement after labor

sarc-   flesh / fleshy material

Examples:
- sarcolysis (sarc/o/lysis)—disintegration of the soft tissues; disintegration of flesh
- sarcocele (sarc/ o/cele)—any fleshy swelling
- sarcoma, -sarcoma (sarc/oma, -sarc/oma)—a tumor made up of fleshy substance
- adenochondrosarcoma (aden/o/chondr/o/sarc/oma)—a tumor containing the elements of adenoma, chondroma and sarcoma, that is a tumor blended of glandular, cartilaginous and fleshy substances

somni-   sleep

Examples:
- somnipathy (somni/path/y)—any disorder of sleep; a hypnotic trance
- somniferous (somni/ fer/ous)—inducing or causing sleep (-*ferous* is an ending meaning "producing")
- insomnia (in/somn/ia)—inability to sleep; also called hypo/somn/ia
- hypersomnia (hyper/somn/ia)—"excessive sleep"; uncontrollable drowsiness; abnormally excessive sleep
- somnolence (somnol/ence)—sleepiness

spas-   pull; draw / contraction

A form of this root -*spasm,* was learned in Lesson 1 with the meaning "involuntary contraction." The root *spas-* indicates any of the involuntary muscular movements ranging in severity from mild but annoying muscle twitches through cramps to convulsion.

-spasia (-spas/ia)—a condition of muscular contraction:

- myospasia *(my/o/spas/ia)*—a spasmodic condition in which rigidity of the muscles is followed immediately by relaxation

-spasmia (-spasm/ia)—a disease characterized by spasms:

- myospasmia (my/o/spasm/ ia)—disease characterized by uncontrollable muscle spasms

spastic (spast/ic)—of the nature of or characterized by spasms

tens-   stretch

The key to this element lies in the root *ten-* that carries a basic meaning of "stretch" and is applied in medical terminology to convey the idea of "stretcher" (a thing that stretches) or "stretching" (the act, or action, of extending or reaching out). The root appears in several forms:

- tensor (tens/or)—any muscle that stretches, or tenses, some part of the body
- tension (tens/ion)—the act or condition of being stretched or strained
  - muscular tension (tens/ion)—the condition of moderate tension produced by stretching a muscle
  - neurotension (neur/o/tens/ion)—the surgical stretching of a nerve
- tendon (tend/on)—any of the cords of tough, fibrous connective tissue which muscle fibers end and by which muscles are attached to bones or other parts

teno-, tenono-, tenonto- (ten/o, tenon/o-, tenont/o)—forms denoting relationship to tendons:

- tenotomy (ten/otomy)—the cutting of a tendon
- tenonitis or tenontitis (tenon/itis, tenont/itis)— inflammation of a tendon

thel-   nipple / a thin layer of tissue

Primarily the root denotes a nipple or teat.

Examples:
- thelium (thel/ium)—name for the nipple
- thelitis (thel/itis)—inflammation of the nipple

The meaning of the root has been extended in the suffix combination -*thelium* that denotes a tissue forming a covering or lining of a body surface.

- epithelium (epi/thel/ium)—a tissue covering surfaces, forming glands, and lining most cavities of the body
- endothelium (end/o/thel/ium)—the layer of cells (tissue) lining the inside of blood and lymph vessels, of the heart, and some other closed cavities

---

thromb-   lump; clot / a thickening; coagulation

This root is principally applied to the clotting properties and problems of the blood.

Examples:

- thrombus (thromb/us)—a clot in a blood vessel or one of the cavities of the heart, formed by coagulation of the blood
- thrombin (thromb/in)—a substance in the blood which helps the blood to clot (such as in a wound)
- thrombosis (thromb/osis)—the formation of a blood clot in a blood vessel or organ
- thrombocyte (thromb/o/cyte)—"a clotting cell"; a small cell in the body which plays an important part in clotting

---

tumor   swelling; mass

A circumscribed, usually non-inflammatory, swelling or mass of new tissue growth arising from existing tissue but developing independently of that tissue's normal rate and structure.

You have learned that *tumor* is the meaning of the elements *-oma*, taught in Lesson 1, and *onco-*, taught in Lesson 5. The use of the word has been covered in the Reading Assignments for both. Tumor is included in this lesson to provide you the way of remembering that it means swelling.

---

vestibule   entrance; a space or cavity around or forming the entrance to a canal or other space

Examples:

- vestibular (vestibul/ar)—pertaining to a vestibule
- vestibule of the mouth—that portion of the oral cavity (cavity of the mouth) between the inside of the lips and cheeks and the outside of the teeth and gums
- buccal vestibule—that portion of the vestibule of the mouth which lies between the inside of the cheeks and the outside of the teeth and gums
- labial vestibule—that portion of the vestibule of the mouth which lies between the inside of the lips and the outside of the teeth and gums
- vestibular labyrinth—pertaining to one of two chambers of the inner ear known as the labyrinth

Lesson 11—Element Recognition

Separate the word terminals, elements, and connecting vowels of the following medical terms from right to left by inserting a slash mark (/) between them.

Example: vestibuloplasty—vestibul/o/plast/y

thrombocyst	sarcomyces
ablactation	macroesthesia
phrenoplegia	laloplegia
theleplasty	intraosseous
exenteritis	interchondral
tumorigenesis	infrapsychic
vestibulotomy	cryalgesia
sarcadenoma	glomoid
prolific	somnific
macronychia	pharmacomania
laloneurosis	lumbodynia
intraleukocyte	thrombogenesis
interpalpebral	ablepharia
infracostal	paraplegia
cryesthesia	thelalgia
malpractice	exodontia
glomangioma	lienocele
hypertension	inframaxillary
somnipathy	lumbodorsal
pharmacodynamics	lienorenal
lumbocostal	lalophobia

Lesson 11—Interpretation Exercise

Complete the following statements by printing the meanings of the elements that make up the medical term in the proper blanks. (Remember, most medical terms are interpreted from right to left.)

11-1.   The word abnormal (ab/normal) means _____ _____ normal.

11-2.   Antepartum (ante/part/um) denotes occurring _____ _____.

11-3.   The term hematocryal (hemat/o/cry/al) means _____ _____.

11-4.   The term exogenic (exo/gen/ic) means _____ _____.

11-5.   A glomus (glom/us) is a _____ _____ anatomical swelling made up of tiny blood vessels.

11-6.   Inframammary (infra/mamm/ary) refers to being situated _____ the _____ gland.

11-7.   Intermuscular (inter/muscul/ar) denotes being _____ _____.

11-8.   Intraspinal (intra/spin/al)denotes being situated or occurring _____ the _____ column.

11-9.   Lalopathy (lal/o/path/y) denotes any _____ of _____.

11-10. Lien is the medical name for the _____.

11-11. The term lumbar (lumb/ar) pertains to the _____.

11-12. The term macrophthalmia (macr/ophthalm/ia) means _____ _____.

11-13. Maldigestion (mal/digestion) denotes _____ digestion.

11-14. Photopharmacology (phot/o/pharmac/ology) is the _____ of the effects of

_____ and other radiations on _____.

11-15. Panplegia (pan/plegia) is a term that means _____ _____.

11-16. The term proliferous (proli/fer/ous) denotes being characterized by the production

of _____.

11-17. The term puerile (puer/ile) means pertaining to _____.

11-18. A sarcoma (sarc/oma) is a tumor made up of _____ substance.

11-19. Somnipathy (somni/pathy) is any _____ of _____.

11-20. Myospasmia (my/o/spasm/ia is a condition characterized by uncontrollable

_____ _____.

11-21. A tensor (tens/or) is any muscle that _____ some part of the body.

11-22. Thelium (thel/ium) is the medical name for the _____.

11-23. A thrombocyte (thromb/o/cyte) is a _____ _____.

11-24. The word tumor means _____.

11-25. The term vestibular (vestibul/ar) means pertaining to an _____.

Lesson 12

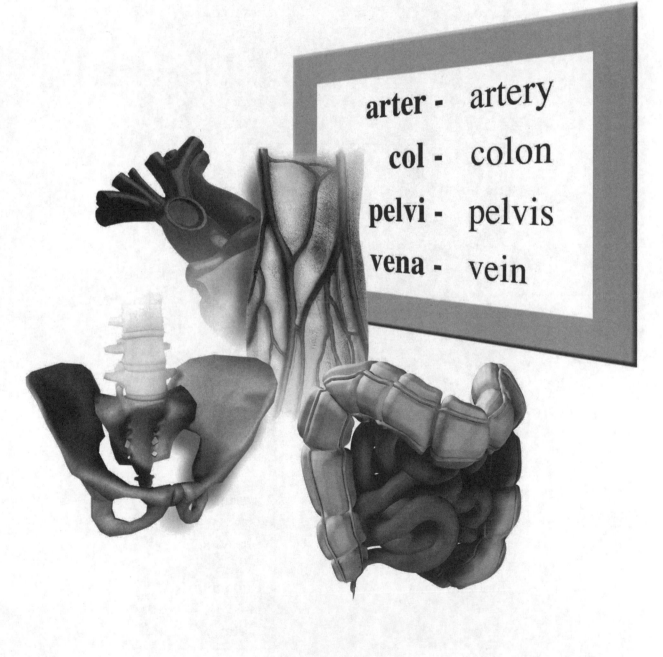

arter - artery
col - colon
pelvi - pelvis
vena - vein

Lesson 12—Review

You will recognize the meanings of all the elements taught in this lesson (or, after seeing them you will know their meanings). Therefore, no audionyms or associations are necessary.

Element	Meaning
arter-	artery
appendic-	appendix
thyro-	thyroid
splen-	spleen
ovario-	ovary
adreno-	adrenal (gland)
basi-	base
pelvi-	pelvis
vena-	vein
urethr-	urethra
utero-	uterus
sacro-	sacrum
pharyng-	pharynx
duodeno-	duodenum
ureter-	ureter

Lesson 12—Review

Element		Meaning
laryng-		larynx
bronch-		bronchus
col-		colon
esophag-		esophagus
bi-		two, double, both
tri-		three
ile-*		ileum
ili-*		ilium
lig-		ligament
therap-		therapy

*Be careful to distinguish between, "*ile- (ileum)*" the lowest part of the small intestine and, "*ili-(ilium)*" the uppermost portion of the three sections of the hipbone. Use the following memory aids to distunguish them:

The "e" ending in, "*ile-*" relates to the "e" in "enter" (intestines).
The "i" ending in, "*ili-*" relates to the "i" in "hip."

Complete the following:

Element	Meaning
arter-	_____
appendic-	_____
thyro-	_____
splen-	_____
ovario-	_____
adreno-	_____
basi-	_____
pelvi-	_____
vena-	_____
urethr-	_____
utero-	_____
sacro-	_____
pharyng-	_____
duodeno-	_____
ureter-	_____
laryng-	_____
bronch-	_____
col-	_____
esophag-	_____
bi-	_____
tri-	_____
ile-	_____
ili-	_____
lig-	_____
therap-	_____

adreno- adrenal gland

The "near or toward the kidney" glands; either of a pair of endocrine ("secreting within") glands lying immediately above the kidney, producing a variety of hormones.

Examples:
- adrenal (adren/al)—situated near the kidney; an adrenal gland
- adrenogenous (adren/o/gen/ous)—produced or arising in the adrenal glands
- adrenalopathy (adren/al/o/path/y)—any disease of the adrenal glands; also called adrenopathy

appendic- appendix

An outgrowth of an organ, especially a small, saclike appendage extending from the large intestine that is commonly called "the appendix" but is technically termed the vermiform appendix (the element *vermi-* means "worm," therefore, because of its shape, "the worm-shaped appendix"). See *scol-* in Reading Assignment of Lesson 14.

A patient may have appendic/e/algia (or append/algia) accompanied by appendic/itis that is relieved by the performance of an append/ectomy.

Example:
- appendiceal (appendic/e/al)—pertaining to an appendix; also appendic/ul/ar

arter- artery

Any one of the system of large, thick-walled tubes that carry blood directly from the heart to the principal parts of the body (as opposed to a vein that carries blood back to the heart).

Examples:
- arterial (arter/ial)—pertaining to an artery or the arteries
- arteriectasis (arteri/ectasis)—dilatation of an artery
- arteriectopy (arteri/ec/top/y)—displacement of an artery from its normal location
- arteriosclerosis (arteri/o/scler/osis)—hardening (sclerosis) and thickening of the arteries

basi- base

The thing or part on which something rests; lowest part or bottom; foundation.

Examples:

- basal (bas/al)—pertaining to or situated near a base; fundamental
- basilysis (basi/lysis)—the crushing of the base of the fetal skull to facilitate delivery
- basiotripsy (basi/o/tripsy)—the crushing of the fetal head to facilitate delivery
- basis (bas/is)—the lower, basic, or fundamental of an object; used as a general term to designate the base of a structure, organ, or part opposite to, or distinguished from, the apex (apic-) or tip

bi-   two, double, both, pair

Also twice, doubly, in pairs.

Examples:

- bigeminy (bi/gemin/y)—the condition of occurring in pairs such as the occurrence of two beats of the pulse in rapid succession
- bipedal (bi/ped/al)—with, or pertaining to, both feet
- birhinia (bi/rhin/ia)—double nose
- biramus (bi/ramus)—consisting of or possessing two branches

This prefix may also appear in the form *bin-* meaning "two" or "both":

- binaural (bin/aur/al)—pertaining to both ears; also bin/ot/ic
- binocular (bin/ocul/ar)—pertaining to both eyes

bronch-   bronchus

Either of the two main branches from the trachea or windpipe that carry air into the lungs. The plural of bronchus (that is, the left bronchus and right bronchus taken together) is bronchi. The point at which the bronchi branch from the trachea is named the tracheal bifurcation (furca, Lesson 8).

Examples:

- bronchial (bronch/i/al)—pertaining to the bronchi
- bronchitis (bronch/itis)—inflammation of the bronchial tubes
- bronchopneumonia (bronch/o/pneumon/ia)—a name given to an inflammation of the lungs, which usually begins in the end of the bronchi
- bronchopleuropneumonia (bronch/o/pleur/o/pneumon/ia)—pneumonia complicated by bronchitis and pleurisy

col-   colon

The largest section of the large intestine.

Examples:

- colic (col/ic)—pertaining to the colon; also used to denote acute abdominal pain

- colocentesis (col/o/centesis)—surgical perforation (puncture) of the colon; also called col/i/puncture and col/o/puncture
- colopexy (col/o/pexy)—fixation of a bend of the colon to the abdominal wall
- colopexotomy (col/o/pex/otomy)—fixation and incision of the colon

duodeno- duodenum

The first section of the small intestine immediately following the stomach.

Examples:
- duodenal (duoden/al)—of, pertaining to, or situated in the duodenum
- duodenocholangeitis (duoden/o/chol/ange/itis)—inflammation of the duodenum and common bile duct
- duodenocholecystostomy (duoden/o/chole/cyst/ostomy)—surgical creation of an opening (communication) between the gallbladder and the duodenum

esophag- esophagus

The tube through which food passes from the pharynx to the stomach; the gullet.

☞ **Note:** *esophag-* is a combination of two elements, the prefix *eso-* meaning "inner, inward" and *phage* (Lesson 8) meaning "to eat" (swallow); just as the mouth and throat provide the "outer swallowing" of food destined for digestion in the stomach, the esophagus takes care of the "inner swallowing," the final stage of passing food to the stomach.

Examples:
- esophageal (esophag/e/al)—pertaining to or belonging to the esophagus
- esophagoptosis (esophag/o/ptosis)—prolapse (falling down or downward displacement of the esophagus)
- esophagocele (esophag/o/cele)—abnormal distention of the esophagus; hernia of the esophagus; protrusion of the mucous and submucous coats of the esophagus through a rupture in the muscular coat, producing a pouch or sac
- esophagomyotomy (esophag/o/my/otomy)—incision through the muscular coat of the esophagus

ile- ileum

The lowest part of the small intestine, opening into the large intestine:
- ileal (ile/al)—pertaining to the ileum
- ileocystoplasty (ile/o/cyst/o/plast/y)—suture of a segment of the ileum to the urinary bladder to increase the bladder size and capacity
- ileoileostomy (ile/o/ile/ostomy)—surgical creation of an opening between two parts of the ileum

ili-   ilium

The flat, uppermost portion of the three sections of the hipbone.

Examples:
- iliac (ili/ac)—pertaining to the ilium
- iliocostal (ili/o/cost/al)—pertaining to the ilium and the ribs
- iliolumbocosto-abdominal (ili/o/lumb/o/cost/o-abdomin/al)—pertaining to the iliac, lumbar, costal and abdominal regions

laryng-   larynx

The structure of muscle and cartilage just below the pharynx. It helps to form what is commonly termed the "Adam's apple." It acts in three ways: (1) as a passage-way for air to the lungs; (2) as an aid in swallowing; (3) as the "voice box," that is the container of the vocal cords which aid in the formation of sounds.

Examples:
- laryngeal (laryng/e/al)—of or pertaining to the larynx
- laryngology (laryng/ology)—that branch of medicine that has to do with the throat. Although, technically, the larynx is only part of the throat, laryngology embraces all parts of the throat. The throat can be described as that part of the neck in front of the spinal column, including the passage through it. It contains the pharynx, the larynx, the trachea and the upper part of the esophagus.
- otolaryngology (ot/o/laryng/ology)—otology (the study of the ear) and laryngology (the study of the throat) considered as a single specialty
- rhinolaryngology (rhin/o/laryng/ology)—rhinology (the study of the nose) and laryngology considered as a single specialty
- otorhinolaryngology (ot/o/rhin/o/laryng/ology)— otology, rhinology and laryngology considered as a single specialty; also designated by the abbreviation E.N.T.

lig-   ligament

The element *lig-* carries the meanings "tie" or "bind." A lig/ament is a band of tough tissue connecting (tying) bones or holding (binding) organs in place.

Examples:
- ligate (lig/ate)—to bind or tie with a ligature
- ligature (lig/at/ure)—a thread or wire for surgical tying
- ligation (lig/at/ion)—the application of a ligature

ovario-   ovary

Ovary was discussed in Lesson 5 and described as the "egg case"; either of the pair of female reproductive glands producing eggs and sex hormones.

Examples:
- ovarian (ovar/ian)—pertaining to an ovary or the ovaries
- ovarin (ovar/in)—an ovarian hormone
- ovariocentesis (ovari/o/centesis)—puncture of the ovary
- ovarioncus (ovari/onc/us)—a tumor of the ovary
- ovariorrhexis (ovari/o/rrhexis)—rupture of an ovary

pelvi- pelvis

Any basinlike or funnel-shaped structure, specifically the basinlike cavity formed by the ring of bones in the hip or pelvic girdle; it is formed by the hipbone together with the sacrum (the bone before the tailbone), supporting the spinal column and resting upon the legs.

Examples:
- pelvic (pelv/ic)—pertaining to the pelvis
- pelvitherm (pelv/i/therm)—an apparatus for applying heat to the pelvic organs through the vagina
- pelvospondylitis (pelv/o/spondyl/itis)— inflammation of the pelvic portion of the spine
- pelviotomy (pelvi/otomy)—the operation of cutting the pelvis at any point to facilitate delivery

pharyng- pharynx

The pharynx is the muscular and membranous cavity of the digestive tube (digestive system), leading from the mouth and nasal passages to the larynx and esophagus. It is about 12.5 centimeters (five inches) long and serves as a passage for air from the nose and mouth; it also is the passage through which food is swallowed after leaving the mouth.

Examples:
- pharyngeal (pharyng/e/al)—pertaining to the pharynx
- pharyngocele (pharyng/o/cele)—hernial protrusion of a part of the pharynx; also called pharyng/o/ectasis
- pharyngalgia (pharyng/algia)—pain in the pharynx, also called pharyng/odyn/ia
- pharyngomycosis (pharyng/o/myc/osis)—any fungus disease of the pharynx
- pharyngosalpingitis (pharyng/o/salping/itis)—inflammation of the pharynx and the eustachian tube

sacro- sacrum

A thick, triangular bone of the vertebral column; the bone above the "tailbone"; it joins with the hip bones to form the back part of the pelvis.

Examples:
- sacral (sacr/al)—pertaining to the sacrum; the region around the sacrum
- sacrad (sacr/ad)—toward the sacrum or sacral region
- sacroplex (sacr/o/plex)—the plexus (network of nerves) stemming from the sacrum

splen-   spleen

The spleen has already been discussed in Lesson 11 under *lien-*.

Examples:
- splenohepatomegaly (splen/o/hepat/o/megal/y)—enlargement of the spleen and the liver
- splenogenous (splen/o/gen/ous)—produced in or formed by the spleen
- splenokeratosis (splen/o/kerat/osis)—hardening of the spleen
- splenolysis (splen/o/lysis)—destruction of spleen tissue
- laparosplenotomy (lapar/o/splen/otomy)—the operation of making an incision into the side to gain access to the spleen, usually for the purpose of draining a cyst or abscess of the spleen

therap-   therapy

The treatment of disease or of any physical or mental disorder by medical or physical means, usually excluding surgery.

Examples:
- therapeutics (therap/eutics)—the science and art of healing
- therapist (therap/ist)—a person skilled in the treatment of disease

thyro-   thyroid

This element may be used to indicate a part such as a cartilage, artery, nerve, etc., in the region of the thyroid gland. The thyroid gland is a large endocrine gland lying in front of and on either side of the windpipe (the trachea). It secretes a hormone that regulates body growth and metabolism.

Examples:
- thyrochondrotomy (thyro/chondr/otomy)—surgical incision of the thyroid cartilage
- thyrooncus (thyro/oncus)—tumor of the thyroid; goiter
- hypothyroidism (hypo/thyroid/ism)—deficiency of thyroid activity or the condition resulting therefrom; also called hypo/thyroid/osis
- hyperthyroidism (hyper/thyroid/ism)— hyperactivity (excess activity) of the thyroid gland; also called hyper/thyroid/osis
- parathyroid (para/thyroid)—(1) situated beside the thyroid gland; (2) any one of four small glands near the lateral lobes of the thyroid

tri-   three

Having, combining, or involving three; triply, in three ways or directions; three times; every three, every third.

Examples:
- trifurcation (tri/furc/ation)—division into three parts; literally "three forks"
- trilateral (tri/later/al)—pertaining to or having three sides
- trilobate (tri/lob/ate)—having three lobes
- tripod (tri/pod)—having three feet
- triorchidism (tri/orchid/ism)—the condition of having three testes or testicles
- triplegia (tri/plegia)—paralysis of three of the extremities

ureter-   ureter

A tube that carries urine from the kidney to the bladder. Note the important root *ur-* which is contained in both ureter and urethra and means urine, that is, the yellowish liquid waste product secreted by the kidneys.

Examples:
- ureteric, ureteral (ureter/ic, ureter/al)—pertaining to the ureter
- ureterectasis (ureter/ectasis)—distention of the ureter
- ureterocutaneostomy (ureter/o/cutan/e/ ostomy)—surgical creation of an opening of the ureter on the skin, permitting drainage of urine directly to the exterior of the body
- ureterolithotomy (ureter/o/lith/otomy)—the removal of a calculus (stone) from the ureter by incision

urethr-   urethra

The canal through which urine is discharged from the bladder to the outside; in the male, semen is also discharged through the urethra.

Examples:
- urethral (urethr/al)—pertaining to the urethra
- urethrocele (urethr/o/cele)—prolapse (hernia) of the female urethra
- urethroplasty (urethr/o/plasty)—plastic surgery of the urethra; operative repair of a wound or defect in the urethra
- urethrostenosis (urethr/o/sten/osis)— narrowing of the urethra
- urethrostomy (urethr/o/stomy)—the formation of a permanent surgical opening into the urethra

utero-   uterus

The uterus, the hollow, muscular organ in the female that serves to protect and nourish the developing embryo and fetus during pregnancy has already been discussed under *hyster-* (Lesson 2) and *metr-* (Lesson 10); also called the womb.

☞   **Note:** The human organism up to the third month following pregnancy is called an embryo; thereafter, that is, the following six months until birth, it is called a fetus. Both the embryonic and fetal development take place in the uterus (see *blast-* in reading assignment of Lesson 14).

Examples:
- uterolith (uter/o/lith)—a uterine calculus or stone
- uterovesical (uter/o/vesic/al)—pertaining to the uterus and the bladder
- uteropexy (uter/o/pexy)—the fixation of a displaced uterus; hyster/o/pexy
- uteritis (uter/itis)—inflammation of the uterus; metr/itis

vena-	vein

The medical word "vena" is the name given to any blood vessel that carries blood from some part of the body back toward the heart. This word is combined with the vowel "e" and used together with a following descriptive word to name the many veins of the body.

Examples:
- venaecerebri (vena/e/cerebr/i)—veins that drain blood from the brain
- venaecordis (vena/e/cor/dis)—veins of the heart, which drain blood from it
- venaehepaticae (vena/e/hepat/icae)—veins that receive blood from the liver

Note: For diseases, abnormalities and therapeutic procedures, the root *phleb-* is used:
- phlebitis (phleb/itis)—inflammation of a vein(s)

Lesson 12—Element Recognition

Separate the word terminals, elements, and connecting vowels of the following medical terms from right to left by inserting a slash mark (/) between them.

Example: thyrochondrotomy—thyro/chondr/otomy

arteriosclerosis	ileoileostomy
appendicolithiasis	iliocostal
thyroaplasia	thermotherapy
splenocele	sacrolumbar
ovariorrhexis	pharyngocele
adrenomegaly	ureterostenosis
basicranial	laryngorhinology
pelvospondylitis	basilateral
venectasia	pelvitherm
urethrocystitis	urethrorrhaphy
uteroplasty	uterolith
sacrarthrogenic	bronchophony
pharyngoplegia	esophagomycosis
duodenocholedochotomy	tricheiria
ureteronephrectomy	ileocolotomy
laryngocentesis	cryotherapy
bronchopneumopathy	iliolumbar
colostomy	arteriostrepsis
esophagocologastrostomy	thyroptosis
biramous	splenomyelomalacia
tridactylism	ovariosalpingectomy

Complete the following statements by printing the meanings of the elements that make up the medical term in the proper blanks. (Remember, most medical terms are interpreted from right to left.)

12-1.   The term adrenalopathy (adren/al/o/path/y) refers to any _____ of the _____ gland.

12-2.   An appendectomy (append/ectomy) is the surgical _____ of the _____.

12-3.   Arteriosclerosis (arteri/o/scler/osis) refers to a condition of _____ of the _____.

12-4.   The term basal (bas/al) means pertaining to or situated near a _____.

12-5.   The term bipedal (bi/ped/al) means with _____ _____.

12-6.   Bronchitis (bronch/itis) is an _____ of the _____ tubes.

12-7.   The term colocentesis (col/o/centesis) denotes a surgical procedure by which the _____ is _____.

12-8.   A duodenocholecystostomy (duoden/o/chole/cyst/ostomy) is a surgical procedure to create an _____ between the _____ and the _____.

12-9.   The term esophagoptosis (esophag/o/ptosis) denotes a _____ _____ of the _____.

12-10. The term ileal (ile/al) pertains to the _____, the lowest part of the small intestine.

12-11. The term iliac (ili/ac) pertains to the _____, the flat uppermost portion of the three sections of the hipbone.

12-12. The term laryngeal (laryng/e/al) pertains to the _____ however the term laryngology (laryng/ology) denotes the _____ of the entire _____.

12-13. A ligament (lig/ament) is a band of tough tissue that _____ bones or organs in place.

12-14. The term ovariorrhexis (ovari/o/rrhexis) denotes a _____ of an _____.

12-15. Pelviotomy (pelvi/otomy) is a surgical procedure of _____ the _____ at any point to facilitate delivery.

12-16. Pharyngalgia (pharyng/algia) denotes _____ in the _____.

12-17. The term sacral (sacr/al) denotes pertaining to, of, or the region around the _____.

12-18. The term splenohepatomegaly (splen/o/hepat/o/megal/y) denotes an _____ of the _____ and _____.

12-19. Therapy is the treatment of a physical or mental disorder by medical or _____ means.

12-20. The term hyperthyroidism (hyper/thyroid/ism) indicates a condition of having _____ activity of the _____ gland.

12-21. Triorchidism (tri/orchid/ism) indicates a condition of having _____ _____.

12-22. The term ureteric (ureter/ic) pertains to the _____, the tube that carries _____ from the kidney to the bladder.

12-23. Urethrostenosis (urethr/o/sten/osis) denotes a _____ of _____ of the _____.

12-24. Uteritis (uter/itis) and also metritis (metr/itis) refers to an _____ of the _____.

12-25. The vena cava inferior is the large _____ entering and returning blood to the heart from the lower extremities and regions of the body.

—Lesson 13*—

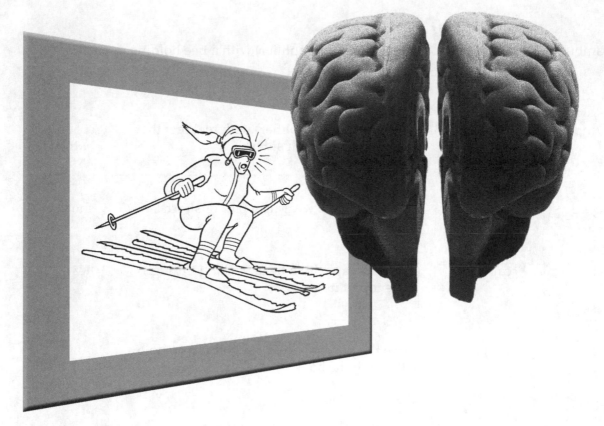

Lessons 13 and 14 including the Reference Section focuses on the diseases and operations of the major body systems

*Formerly Lesson II-1

Lesson 13—Review

Element	Audionym	Visual Image	Meaning
ventr-	vent	See the **vent** with the **front** of a man in it!	front
vert-	vertebrae	See the **vert**ebrae that **turn**s and **turn**s!	turn
eu-	ukulele	See the **u**kulele being eaten because it tastes so **good**!	good
ambi-	amp bee	See the **amp** (amplifier) with a **be**e holding a phone **booth**!	both
amphi-	amp feet	See the **amp** (amplifier) with real **fee**t that are **round** on **both sides**!	around, on both sides
brachy-	brake	See the **brake** wearing a pair of **short**s!	short
capit-	cap	See the **cap** with a **head** sticking through the top of it!	head
cau-	cough	See the person whose **cou**gh **burn**s a hole through the book!	burn
clas-	class	See the **clas**s (of students) that **break**s in half!	break
duct-	duck	See the **duc**k with a **tube** around its neck!	tube
fiss-	fish	See the **fis**h that's **split**!	split

Element	Audionym	Visual Image	Meaning
ger-	jar	See the **jar** with an **old** man in it!	old
heter-	header	See the **header** with an **udder** on it!	other
infer-	inn fur	See the "**inn fur**" (an **inn** made of **fur**) **under** water!	under
hom-	home	See the **hom**e changed into many **hom**es that look the **same**!	same
olfact-	oil factory	See the **oil fact**ory with a terrible **smell**!	smell
orth-	Orthodox (Church)	See the **Orth**odox Church with workers trying to make it **straight**!	straight
gyn-	gun, gin	See the **gun** shaped like a bottle of **gin** with a **female** coming out of it!	female
pachy-	pack	See the back**pack** become very **thick**!	thick
phrag-	fur rag	See the **fur rag** with a **fence** coming out of it!	fence
poster-	poster	See the **poster** with people looking at the **back part** of it!	back part
cata-	catalog	See the **cat**alog with **down** all over it!	down
platy-	plate	See the **plate** so **flat** that the food slides off it!	flat
pseud-	suit	See the **suit** with **false** teeth on it!	false
schiz-	skis	See the **skis** that **split**!	split

Substitute this page for use with all previous program editions

Lesson 13—Worksheet

Print the audionym and meaning of the elements in the proper blanks:

Element	Audionym	Meaning
ventr-		
vert-		
eu-		
ambi-		
amphi-		
brachy-		
capit-		
cau-		
clas-		
duct-		
fiss-		
ger-		
heter-		
infer-		
hom-		
olfact-		
orth-		
gyn-		
pachy-		
phrag-		
poster-		
cata-		
platy-		
pseud-		
schiz-		

Lesson 13—Reading Assignment

ambi-, ambo-   sometimes amb-, am-, an- —both, on both sides, around

You may know that ambi/dextrous means equal ease in using both hands. If you know that an introvert (intro/vert; inner turning) is a person whose thoughts and concerns are directed mostly within himself; that an extrovert (outer turning) is a person whose thoughts and concerns are directed principally toward others, then it would follow that an ambivert (ambi/vert) would have both "inner turning" and "outer turning" characteristics.

Examples:
- ambisexual (ambi/sexual)—pertaining to or affecting both sexes
- ambient (ambi/ent)—surrounding, on both or all sides
- amplexation (am/plex/ation)—braid or weave around

amphi-, ampho-   both, in two ways; roundabout, around

An amphitheater (amphi/theater) is an oval or U-shaped structure surrounded by rows of seats. An amphibian (amphi/bi/an) can maintain life (*bi-, bio-*) in two environments. Some frogs and snakes are equally at home on water or land and are classified as amphi/bi/ans. Aircraft and tanks or other vehicles that can travel on either land or water are called amphi/bi/ans.

Examples:
- amphicrania (amphi/cran/ia)—pain on both sides of the head
- amphodiplopia (amph/o/dipl/op/ia)—double vision in both eyes

brachy-   short

- brachyfaci/al (brachy/faci/al)—low, broad face
- brachygnathia (brachy/gnath/ia)—abnormal shortness of the underjaw
- brachycheilia (brachy/cheil/ia)—shortness of the lip
- brachymorphic (brachy/morph/ic)—built along lines that are shorter than those of the normal figure
- brachymetropia (brachy/metr/op/ia)—nearsightedness

capit-   (cep, cip-) head

You learned in Lesson 3 that cephal- means "head." *Capit-*, sometimes abbreviated to *cep-* or *cip-* also means "head." You may recognize the figurative use of *capit-* in capital (capit/al) "pertaining to the head." In the case of capit/al we mean the "head of government."

Examples:
- capitopedal (capit/o/ped/al)—pertaining to the head and foot
- decapitate (de/capit/ate)—"head from"; the act of beheading
- occipital (oc/cipit/al)—"back of head"; pertaining to the back of the head
- occipital bone (oc/cipit/al bone)—the bone that forms the back of the skull
- biceps (bi/cep/s)—"two-headed"; a muscle having two heads or points of origin; especially the large muscle in the front of the upper arm or the corresponding muscle at the back of the thigh

cata-, cath-; (kath-) down, under, lower; complete

A catastrophe (cata/stroph/e) is a complete failure or extreme "downturning." A cate/gory is lower or less than the whole. A cata/log is a complete written list.

Examples:
- catarrh (cata/rrh)—(rrh is an abbreviated form of rrhe-) a "flowing down"; inflammation of a mucous membrane with a discharge of mucus
- catalyst (cata/lys/t)—a "loosening down"; a substance which speeds up, or sometimes slows down, the rate of a chemical reaction
- catheter (cath/et/er)—a "sending down"; a slender tube which is inserted into a body cavity

cau-, caus-, caut-, caust- burn, burning heat
cauter- a searing or burning, such as with a hot iron

You may know that lye, sulphuric acid, or other chemicals that destroy or eat away are called caustic (caust/ic) substances. Or perhaps you have heard someone described as having a caust/ic wit, that is, a "burning" or destructive manner of commenting.

Examples:
- caustic (caust/ic)—burning or corrosive; destructive to human tissue
- causalgia (caus/alg/ia)—a burning pain
- cauterize (cauter/ize)—the application of a caust/ic substance, a hot iron, an electric current, or other means of killing tissue
- thermocautery (therm/o/cauter/y)—cauter/ization by means of a heated wire or point

-clas-, -clast break, destroy

Examples:
- osteoclasia (oste/o/clas/ia)—the destruction and absorption of bone

-cla/sis the surgical procedure whereby a part, usually a bone, is broken (fractured) or rebroken (refractured) for the purpose of repair or reconstruction:
- osteoclasis (oste/o/cla/sis)—the breaking of a bone to correct a deformity
- osteoclast (oste/o/clast)—an instrument used to perform oste/o/cla/sis
- cardioclasis (cardi/o/cla/sis)—literally a "broken heart"; actually, rupture of the heart

- diaclasis (dia/cla/sis)—a fracture (break through or apart), especially one for a surgical purpose

duct- a tube, a channel or canal through which a substance moves: also, *"duct-"* means to lead or draw

Examples:

- ductless glands (duct/less glands)—glands producing internal secretions that are introduced directly into the bloodstream (rather than through a duct) for transport to the rest of the body:
  - The thyroid, adrenal, and pituitary glands are ductless (duct/less) or endocrines (end/o/crin/e/s)

In your home you may have a heating duct which is a tube that carries heated air from the furnace to each room. An aqueduct is a tube or channel that carries water. An orchestra con/duct/or or a tour con/duct/or is a leader. An ab/duct/or is one who leads or draws (actually forces) another away.

Examples:

- abduct (ab/duct)—to draw away from the midline of the body; an instance would be the raising of the arm outward and to the side:
  - abductor (ab/duct/or)—a muscle that draws a part of the body away from the midline
  - adductor (ad/duct/or)—the opposite of ab/duct/or; a muscle that draws a part of the body toward the midline

eu- good, well; normal; easy

You may be familiar with a eulogy (eu/log/y), "good speaking," a formal speech praising a person who has recently died; euthanasia (eu/thanas/ia), "good death" (*thanas-* is an element meaning death), that has been advocated by some as a way to deal with persons dying of incurable, painful diseases.

Examples:

- The element *eu-* is used in medical terms to indicate normal functioning in the form eu/_____/ia:
- eucholia (eu/chol/ia)—normal bile
- euglcyemia (eu/glyc/em/ia)—normal level of glucose in the blood
- eukinesia (eu/kines/ia)—normal movement
- eupnea (eu/pne/a)— normal breathing, normal respiration

fiss-, fid- to split, cleave

Nuclear fisson (fiss/ion), the splitting of atomic particles to produce nuclear energy, is currently a matter of great public concern.

Examples:

- fissure (fiss/ure)—any cleft or groove, normal or otherwise
- fission (fiss/ion)—a splitting apart; a division into parts
- fissula (fiss/ul/a)—a little cleft
- fissura (fiss/ura)—a general term for a cleft or groove; used in anatomical nomenclature to designate the major fiss/ure/s of the body

ger-, geron-, geront- old (in the sense of old age or an old person)

Examples:

- geriatrics (ger/iatr/ics)—the branch of medicine that deals with the diseases and hygiene of old age
- gerontology (geront/ology)—the scientific study of the process of aging and the problems of aged people
- acrogeria (acr/o/ger/ia)—"old extremities"; condition of premature aging of the skin of the hands and feet

gyn-, gynec- female, woman

We're familiar with monogamy (mono/gamy; *-gamy* means marriage) as meaning being married to only one person at a time and poly/gamy as meaning being married to many (that is, more than one) persons at one time. Monogyny (mono/gyn/y) means being married to one woman at a time; polygyny (poly/gyn/y) means being married to many women at one time.

Examples:

- gynecology (gynec/ology)—the branch of medicine dealing with the specific functions and diseases of women. The specialist is a gynec/ologist.
- gynecoid (gynec/oid)—"female-like"; of or characteristic of a woman or women
- gynecomastia (gynec/o/mast/ia)—"woman-breasted condition"; excessive development of the male mammary glands

heter-, hetero-, (-eter-) other, different from (opposite of *homo-*)

To be heterosexual (heter/o/sexual) is to have sexual interest in those of the other or opposite sex.

Examples:

- heterogenous (heter/o/gen/ous)—differing or opposite in structure, quality, etc.
- heterotopia (heter/o/top/ia)—"different place"; displacement or misplacement of parts or organs
- heterodermic (heter/o/derm/ic)—pertaining to a skin graft taken from one of a different species
- myeleterosis (myel/eter/osis)—morbid alteration of the spinal cord

hom-, homo-, homeo-   same, the same, equal; like, resembling (as opposed to heter- "different")

☞   **Note:** The word homo also refers to the biological class that includes modern man, as well as manlike mammals such as apes and monkeys; within this class modern man is further classified as homo sapiens, "the wise one."

A homosexual (homo/sexual) is one who has a sexual preference for those of the same sex. Homogenized (homo/gen/ized) milk has been processed so that cream (the fat element) is so finely divided and emulsified as not to separate.

Examples:

- homogenous (hom/o/gen/ous)—"standing the same"; a tendency toward uniformity or stability in the normal body states
- homohemotherapy (homo/hem/o/therapy)—treatment by the injection of blood from another individual of the same species
- homeotransplant (home/o/trans/plant)—a piece of tissue taken from one individual and transplanted in another individual of the same species

infer-   below

We have a sense of the meaning "lower" or "below" in our use of the word "inferior" (infer/ior):

- inferior (infer/ior)—situated below or located downward

The combining form infero (infer/o-) denotes "below and":

- inferolateral (infer/o/later/al)—situated below and to one side
- inferomedian (infer/o/med/ian)—situated in the middle of the underside
- inferoposterior (infer/o/poster/ior)—situated below and behind

olfact-   smell; to smell

Examples:

- olfaction (olfact/ion)—the act of smelling; the sense of smell
- olfactophobia (olfact/o/phob/ia)—morbid aversion to odors
- olfactory (olfact/ory)—pertaining to the sense of smell

orth-, ortho-   straight; correct, normal

The applications of *orth-* in medical terms are related to our common usage of the word "straight." Straight can be used in the sense of the same direction throughout, as in "a straight line." In expressions such as "going straight" and "straighten out" we are using "straight" in the sense of "normal" or "correct."

Examples:

- anorthopia (an/orth/op/ia)—"not straight vision"; distorted vision
- orthosis (orth/osis)—the straightening of a distorted part
- orthuria (orth/ur/ia)—normal frequency of urination

Most medical terms using *ortho-* carry the meaning "correction of deformity" or "correction of malfunction":

Examples:

- orthodontics (orth/odont/ics)—the branch of dentistry concerned with correcting and preventing irregularities of the teeth and poor "bite"
- orthopedics (orth/o/ped/ics)—the branch of surgery dealing with the treatment of deformities, diseases, and injuries of the bones, joints, muscles, etc. [*ped-* refers to child since many deformities and malfunctions are congenital (con/genit/al), "born together"; that is, existing at birth; however, orthopedics is not confined to children]

---

pachy-   thick

Have you ever heard an elephant referred to as a pachy/derm? Actually, any large, thickskinned animal such as an elephant, a rhinoceros, or a hippopotamus is a pachy/derm.

Examples:

- pachydermia (pachy/derm/ia)—skin thickness; abnormal thickness of the skin
- pachyemia (pachy/em/ia)—blood thickness; thickening of the blood
- acropachy (acr/o/pach/y)—clubbed (thickened) fingers and toes

---

phrag-, phrax-   to fence in, wall off, block up

Examples:

- diaphragm (dia/phrag/m)—"blocking across"; a partition; the partition of muscles and tendons between the chest cavity and the abdominal cavity; the midriff
- urethrophraxis (urethr/o/phrax/is)—blocking (obstruction) of the urethra
- kataphraxis (kata/phrax/is)—the operation to enclose or surround an organ with metal supports (a fencing in) to keep it in place

---

platy-   broad, flat
plak-, plax-, plat-   flat or broad like a plate; a patch of eruption

We use plate, platform, plane, platter (not only as a utensil but to describe a phonograph record). All of these words contain the impression of flatness. A plain (as in the Great Plains) carries the idea of breadth and flatness.

Examples:
- The form platy/_____/ia or platy/_____/ic—is used to describe broadness or flatness in many body parts, platy/pod/ia—flatfooted; abnormal flatness of the feet
- The form -plak/ia— indicates abnormal patches, as on the skin, mucous membrane, etc.
- leukoplakia (leuk/o/plak/ia)—the development of white patches upon the tissues of the mouth
- malacoplakia (malac/o/plak/ia)—the formation of soft patches on mucous membranes such as those of the bladder and ureters

poster-   back part, behind

☞ **Note:** As you probably suspect, this element is related to the element *post-* meaning after or behind.

Example:
- posterior (poster/ior)—at or toward the rear

postero- (poster/o-)—behind and_____; situated behind and_____:
- posteroinferior (poster/o/infer/ior)—behind and below
- posterosuperior (poster/o/super/ior)—behind and above
- posterolateral (poster/o/later/al)—behind and to one side

pseud-   false, imaginary; like in appearance but unlike in structure or function

You may know that a pseudonym (pseud/o/nym) is a "false name," that is, a fictitious name or pen name used by an author who does not want her real name to be known. In medical terms *pseud-* is used to indicate something that looks like or has the outward appearance of one thing but, in basic structure or the way it performs, it is not the thing it appears to be.

Example:
- pseudopregnancy (pseud/o/pregnancy)—false pregnancy

The root may appear in the form pseud/__ /ia or pseud/__ /osis, indicating symptoms characteristic of one condition, but actually arising from some other (frequently less serious) cause:
- pseudesthesia (pseud/esthesia)—"false feeling"; sensations that are felt without the usual accompanying causes or stimulus
- pseudocirrhosis (pseud/o/cirrh/osis)—apparent cirrh/osis of the liver due to some other cause

    pseud/o/_____/itis—"false inflammation"
    pseud/o/_____/oma—"false tumor"

schiz- (schis-)   split

Examples:
- schizophrenia (schiz/o/phren/ia)—"split mind"; a major mental disorder typically characterized by a separation (split) between the thought processes and the emotions
- cheiloschisis (cheil/o/schis/is)—"split lip"; harelip
- schizonychia (schiz/onych/ia)—splitting of the nails

ventr-, ventro-   front/also, belly, abdomen, cavity

Examples:
- ventral (ventr/al)—the front of the body; the belly side; the abdominal region; opposed to dors/al
- ventricle (ventr/icle)—"little cavity"; small cavities or pouches; the heart

ventro- (ventr/o-)—the belly or front and_____; the front part of_____:
- ventrodorsad (ventr/o/dors/ad)—from the ventr/al (front) toward the dors/al (back)
- ventrocystorrhapy (ventr/o/cysto/rrhaphy)—the stitching (suturing) of a cyst; or the stitching of the bladder to the abdominal wall

vert-, vers-   to turn, a turn

Examples:
- vertebra (vert/ebra)—any of the single bones or segments of the spinal column; the arrangement of bones that permits us to turn or twist our bodies
- version (vers/ion)—a displacement (turning) of the uterus; also, the operation of turning the fetus during childbirth
- vertigo (vert/igo)—a sensation of dizziness in which we feel that we or our surrounding is turning or whirling about in a sickening manner
- transverse (trans/vers/e)—"turned across"; placed crosswise; situated at a right angle to the long axis of a body or organ
- retroversion (retro/vers/ion)—"turned back"; the tipping of an entire organ backward

Lesson 13—Element Recognition

Separate the word terminals, elements, and connecting vowels of the following medical terms from right to left by inserting a slash mark (/) between them.

ambilateral

amphicarcinogenic

brachycephalic

capitate

cataplasia

diaclasia

ductal

euesthesia

subfissure

geroderma

gynopathy

heterodont

homodont

inferior

olfactology

orthodontics

pachyderm

diaphragm

platypodia

posterior

pseudoesthesia

schizophrenia

ventral

invert

Lesson 13—Interpretation Exercise

Complete the following statements by printing the meanings of the elements that make up the medical term in the proper blanks. (Remember, most medical terms are interpreted from right to left.)

13-1.   The term ambisexual (ambi/sexual) denotes pertaining to _____ sexes.

13-2.   The term amphipod (amphi/pod) denotes having _____ on_____ sides.

13-3.   The term brachycheilia (brachy/cheil/ia) denotes a _____ _____.

13-4.   The term capitopedal (capit/o/ped/al) pertains to the _____ and _____.

13-5.   A catalyst (cata/lys/t) is a substance that speeds up or _____ the rate of chemical change.

13-6.   The term causalgia (caus/algia) denotes a _____ _____.

13-7.   Osteoclasis (oste/o/cla/sis) the surgical procedure of _____ a _____ to correct a deformity or make a repair.

13-8.   A duct is a _____ through which gas or liquid flows.

13-9.   The term euglycemia (eu/glyc/em/ia) denotes a _____ level of glucose in the the _____.

13-10. Fission (fiss/ion) is a term that means a _____ apart.

13-11. The term acrogeria (acr/o/ger/ia) refers to_____ _____.

13-12. Gynecoid (gynec/oid) means _____ a _____.

13-13. To be heterosexual (heter/o/sexual) is to have sexual interest in the _____ sex.

13-14. A homosexual (homo/sexual) is one who has a sexual preference for those of the _____ sex.

13-15. Inferolateral (infer/o/later/al) means situated _____ and to the_____.

13-16. The term olfactory (olfact/ory) denotes pertaining to the sense of _____.

13-17. Orthodontics (orth/odont/ics) is the branch of dentistry concerned with_____ and preventing irregularities of the _____ and poor bite.

13-18. Pachyderm (pachy/derm) means _____ _____.

13-19. The term urethrophraxis (urethr/o/phrax/is) denotes a _____ off of the _____ by an obstruction.

13-20. Platypodia (platy/pod/ia) denotes _____ _____.

13-21. Posterosuperior (poster/o/super/ior) denotes being _____ and _____.

13-22. The term pseudopregnancy (pseud/o/pregnancy) means a _____ _____.

13-23. Schizophrenia (schiz/o/phren/ia) which means _____ _____ is a mental disorder typically characterized by a separation between the thought processes and emotions.

13-24. Ventral (ventr/al) is a term pertaining to the _____ of the body.

13-25. A vertebra (vert/ebra) is any of the bones or segments of the spinal column which in its arrangement with the others permits us to _____.

Lesson 14[*]

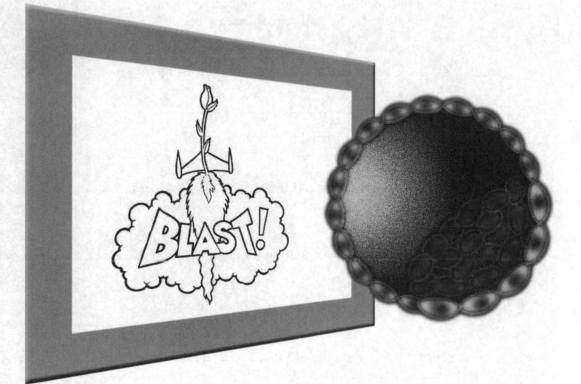

*Formerly Lesson II-2

Lesson 14—Review

Element	Audionym	Visual Image	Meaning
proxim-	peroxide	See the **peroxide** with a **knee** covered with **rust**, sticking out of it!	nearest
scol-	school	See the **school** that is **curved**!	curved
apo-	apple	See the **apple** running **away from** you!	away from
di-	dye	See the **dye** coming out both ends of the bottle to **dye** material **twice**!	twice
dia-	diet pill	See the **die**t pill with a hand **through** it!	through
eury-	urinal	See the **uri**nal that is very **broad**!	broad
pect-	pecked	See the **pecked** tree with a treasure **chest** in it!	chest
necr-	neck	See the **nec**k with a **dead** fish around it!	dead
mi-	mice	See the **mi**ce taking a piano **less**on!	less
morph-	mower roof	See the **mo**wer with a **roof**. It has **form**s flying out of it!	form
dis-	discus	See the **dis**cus falling **apart**!	apart
fac-	factory	See the **fac**tory that **make**s **dew** drops!	make, do
lept-	leopard	See the **leo**pard that is very **slender**!	slender

Lesson 14—Review

Element	Audionym	Visual Image	Meaning
lymph-	limp	See the person **limp**ing because he has **water** and **fluid** strapped to his leg!	watery fluid
meta-	metal (metal cabinet)	See the **metal** cabinet with a **bee yawn**ing inside it!	beyond
-rrhag	raging (raging river)	See the **rag**ing river and balloons **burst**ing with **fort**s inside them!	burst, burst forth
sta-	stand	See the music **stand** with another **stand** on top of it!	stand
ton-	ton (truck)	See the **ton** (truck) being **stretch**ed!	stretch
volv-	valve	See the **valve** with **tea roll**s coming out of it!	to roll
splanchn-	"S" plank	See the **"S" plank** that has an **inner tube** with **organs** on it!	internal organs
-rrhe	reed (reed instrument)	See the **reed** instrument with something **flow**ing out of it!	flow
med-	meat	See the **meat** with a hole in the **middle** of it!	middle
xer-	zero	See the **zero** on the thermometer with a clothes **dry**er bursting out of it!	dry
per-	purr	See the cat that **purr**s **throw out** the whole family!	throughout
blast-	blast	See the space ship **blast**ing off and turning into a **bud**!	bud

Lesson 14—Worksheet

Complete the following:

Element	Audionym	Meaning
proxim-		
scol-		
apo-		
di-		
dia-		
eury-		
pect-		
necr-		
mi-		
morph-		
dis-		
fac-		
lept-		
lymph-		
meta-		
-rrhag		
sta-		
ton-		
volv-		
splanchn-		
-rrhe		
med-		
xer-		
per-		
blast-		

apo-   away from, separation, from; lack

To apo/log/ize is to "speak away." Figuratively we "speak away" or say something that corrects some previous action or words that have given offense to someone.

Examples:
- apophysis (apo/phy/sis)—a "growth away from"; an outgrowth, especially a bony outgrowth
- apogeny (apo/gen/y)—lack of the power to reproduce

blast-   bud, shoot, sprout, embryonic cell

The root *blast-* indicates a relationship to something that is formative on the order of a sprouting seed; more specifically to an embry/o. You probably know that a human in the mother's uterus is called an embry/o. Technically, the human organism in the uterus is called an embry/o during the early stages of pregnancy: the period from one week after conception to the end of the second month. From the third month on it is called a fet/us. In its early stages (about the first week or so) the embry/o consists of increasing layers of cells around a central cavity somewhat in the shape of a hollow sphere. At this stage it is called a blast/ul/a (a little bud).

Examples:
- angioblast (angi/o/blast also called angi/o/derm)—the formative tissue from which blood cells are formed
- lipoblast (lip/o/blast)—a tissue cell that develops into a fat cell; an embry/onic fat cell
- blastoma (blast/oma)—a tumor formed from tissues the same as those in the location in which it arises, as contrasted to a tumor composed of tissues in addition to or other than those in the area from which it develops:
  - angioblastoma (angi/o/blast/oma)—a blood vessel tumor
  - lipoblastoma (lip/o/blast/oma)—a tumor made up of lip/o/blast/s or embry/onic fat cells

di-   twice, double, twofold

Dioxides (di/ox/ide/s) such as carbon dioxide are oxides containing two atoms of oxygen for each molecule.

Examples:
- dimorphic (di/morph/ic)—"double form"; occurring in two distinct forms
- diglossia (di/gloss/ia)—double tongue
- dihysteria (di/hyster/ia)—condition of having a double uterus

dia-   across, through, apart

Diameter (dia/meter) is a straight line passing through a circle, or the measure of such a line.

Examples:

- diarrhea (dia/rrhe/a)—a "flowing through"; an excessive flow of loose matter from the bowels
- dialysis (dia/lysis)—a "loosening apart"; a process by which substances in solution are separated from each other; especially the separation of impurities from the blood during kidney failure
- diaphragm (dia/phrag/m)—a "wall across"; a membrane across the body separating the chest from the abdomen

dis-   apart, away, asunder; opposite of

This prefix is similar to *de-* and is widely used both in medicine and in common English. Sometimes it can mean so far apart as to be the opposite of:

dis/ease—the opposite of being at ease; "not ease"
dis/able—the opposite of being able; "not able"

Sometimes it can mean separation, a "putting away":

- dis/miss—a dis/miss/al (particularly from a job) is a separation
- dissect (dis/sect)—"cut apart"; that is, to cut in many pieces
- dislocation (dis/loc/ation)—"apart or away from its place"; specifically, to dis/place a bone from its correct loc/ation
- disesthesia (dis/esthes/ia)—the "opposite feeling"; dis/comfort

eury-   wide, broad (opposed to *sten-* narrow)

Since the effect of widening or broadening is to increase in size, *eury-* carries the meaning "enlargement" due to widening or broadening.

Examples:

- aneurysm (an/eury/sm)—(frequently changed to an/eur/ism) a sac formed by the local enlargement of the weakened wall of an artery, caused by disease or injury
- procteurysis (proct/eury/sis)—dilatation (widening) of the rectum by an instrument
- eurycephalous (eury/cephal/ous)—having a wide head

fac-, fact-, fic-, fect-   make, to do, cause
fac-, faci-, fici-   face; outer surface; form, figure

We have chosen to discuss these elements together because of their similarity and because of the wide usage that each has.

You are familiar with a facial (faci/al) as a treatment intended to improve the skin of the face. A facade (fac/ade) is the front part of anything, the outer surface. Superficial (super/fici/al) means of or being on the surface; sometimes used figuratively to mean shallow in the sense of the obvious and easily seen rather than the deep and profound.

You are also familiar with a factory in which things are manufactured (manu/fact/ured). (*manu-* means "hand" as in manual (manu/al) training; manual labor. Manufacture originally meant "made by hand" although it has now been extended to mean things made by machinery.) To facilitate (fac/il/it/ate) is to make easy. The faculty (fac/ul/ty) of the schools you have attended or are attending is provided to make or cause easy learning, or, as easy as the subject matter and the student permit. In facilitating the learning process the faculty presents facts (fact/s) (that which was done). A good instructor is both effective (ef/fect/ive) and efficient (ef/fici/ent).

lept- thin, slender

Examples:

- leptochymia (lept/o/chym/ia)—thinness (meagerness) of body fluids
- leptodactyly (lept/o/dactyl/y)—abnormal slenderness of fingers and toes
- leptodermic (lept/o/dermic)—thin skinned

lymph-   watery fluid

One of the major fluids of the body found in all parts of the body. Other major fluids are blood and tissue fluid. Lymph is a pale fluid that bathes the tissues, passes into lymph channels and ducts, and is discharged into the blood.

Examples:

- lymphaden (lymph/aden)—referring to a lymph gland or lymph node.

☞ **Note:** The names "lymph gland" and "lymph node" are synonyms. "Lymph node" is the preferred name although "lymph gland" is widely used.

"node" means "knot"; a knotty swelling or protuberance (A protuberance is something that bulges or sticks out.)

med-, mes, medi-, mesi- middle, intermediate

You may know that a medial (medi/al) strip on a highway is a strip down the middle; that an intermediary (inter/medi/ary) is one who comes in between (that is, takes a middle position) without bias toward either side. In nonmedical English we are inclined to use the prefix *med-* or *mid-* more frequently to designate a middle, the middle, something in between. In medical terminology *mes-* is the more frequently used prefix.

Examples:

- mesentery (mes/enter/y)—a membranous fold attaching the small intestine to the base of the abdominal wall
- mesonasal (mes/o/nas/al)—situated in the middle of the nose
- mesoderm (mes/o/derm)—the middle layer of cells in an embryo from which the skeletal, reproductive, muscular, vascular, connective, etc. tissues develop. Logically enough, the ecto/derm is the outside layer and the endo/derm is the inside layer
- mediastinum (mediastin/um)—"occurring in the middle"; a membranous partition between two cavities of the body; especially the membrane separating the lungs

meta- beyond, change, transformation; after

Examples:

- metabolism (meta/bol/ism)—(*bol-* means to throw) to "throw beyond"; change; all of the physical and chemical changes and processes continuously going on in the body by which growth is achieved and energy released
- metamorphosis (meta/morph/o/sis)—"form change"; change in shape or structure
- metastasis (meta/sta/sis)—a "change in standing or status"; the spread of disease from one part of the body to another
- metaplasia (meta/plas/ia)—"development change"; abnormal change of one type of tissue to another; also, conversion of one tissue into another, as the cartilage of the infant into the bone of the adult

mi-, mio-, meio- less, smaller

We commonly use a variation of this element in the form *min-*. Min/or means lesser in size, amount, number, extent, importance, etc. To di/min/ish is to make less. In subtraction, four min/us two means that four is to be diminished (that is, made less or smaller) by two.

Examples:

-miosis, -meiosis (-mio/sis, -mei/osis)—condition of decrease; disintegration:

- osteomiosis (oste/o/mio/sis)—"bone lessening"; disintegration of a bone

- rhinomiosis (rhin/o/mio/sis)—"nose lessening"; surgery for the reduction of the size of the nose
- miocardia (mio/cardia)—the contraction (squeezing thus lessening) movement of the heart; also called systole

morph- form, shape, figure

Examples:

-morphic, -morphous (-morph/ic, -morph/ous)—having a (specified) shape:
- monomorphous (mono/morph/ous)—"single shape"; existing in one form only; having the same form throughout all stages of development isomorphic (iso/morph/ic)—"equal shape"; having similar or identical structure or form
- amorphous (a/morph/ous)—"no shape"; without definite form; shapeless
- metamorphosis (meta/morph/osis)—change in form, shape, structure, or substance

necr- dead

Examples:
- necrosis (necr/osis)—death of tissue
- necrectomy (necr/ectomy)—the cutting away (excision) of dead material
- necrology (necr/ology)—statistics or records of death

-necrosis (-necr/o/sis)—condition of dead tissue:
- rhinonecrosis (rhin/o/necr/osis)—necr/osis of the nasal bones
- osteonecrosis (oste/o/necr/osis)—necr/osis of a bone

pect-, pector- the chest, thorax; the part of the body enclosed by the ribs

Examples:
- expectorate (ex/pector/ate)—"out of the chest"; to cough and spit out (phlegm, mucus, etc.)
- pectoralgia (pector/algia)—pain in the chest
- angina pectoris (pector/is)—(angina means a choking, a strangling) pain in the chest, sometimes extending to the left arm, caused by a sudden decrease of the blood supply to the heart muscle

per- throughout, through; thoroughly, excessively

Examples:
- peracute (per/acute)—excessively acute or sharp
- pernasal (per/nas/al)—"through the nose"; performed through the nose
- percutaneous (per/cutan/eous)—"through the skin"; performed through the skin as an injection

proxim-   near, nearest

We can describe locations as being "in the proxim/ity of_____" by which we mean "near" or "close to." An ap/proxim/ation is an estimate, something which is close (near) enough for practical purposes.

Examples:
- proximal (proxim/al)—nearest; closer to any point of reference; opposed to dist/al (farthest)
- proximate (proxim/ate)—next or nearest
- proximad (proxim/ad)—toward the proxim/al (nearest) end

-rrhag- (rhag-)   burst forth; burst

Example:
- hemorrhage (hem/o/rrhag/e)—(shortened from hem/o/rrhag/ia) a substantial flow of blood; bleeding

Hemorrhage (hem/o/rrhag/e) fully carries the meaning "blood flow" since it contains the root *hem-*. However, the appearance of the ending *-rrhag/ia* usually carries the meaning "blood flow" from the body part to which it is attached:
- enterorrhagia (enter/o/rrhag/ia)—intestinal blood flow
- metrorrhagia (metr/o/rrhag/ia)—uterine bleeding
- odontorrhagia (odont/o/rrhag/ia)—"tooth bleeding"

-rrhe (rhe-)   to flow

Examples:
- diarrhea (dia/rrhe/a)—"to flow through"; excessive looseness or frequency of bowel movements
- otorrhea (oto/rrhe/a)—"ear flow"; a discharge from the ear
- rheum (rhe/um)—any watery or cata/rrh/al discharge
- catarrh (cata/rrh)—"flow down," shortened from cata/rrhe; inflammation of mucous membrane with a free discharge of mucus; runny (that is, flowing) nose

scol-, scoli-   curved, twisted, crooked

Example:
-scoliosis (-scoli/osis)—condition of curvature, crookedness:
- rachiscoliosis (rach/i/scoli/osis)—curvature of the spine; more frequently shortened to scoli/osis without the preceeding *rachi-*

scolec- —form of *scol-*, denoting relationship to a worm; worm-shaped; can refer to the appendix which has the shape of a worm, as in scolec-tomy, a synonym for the preferred term "append/ectomy."

Example:
- scolecoid (scolec/oid)—worm-shaped

☞ **Note:** There are many appendixes (from ad—to + pend—hang) "hanging to" various body structures. The one most frequently encountered is the worm-shaped (scolec/oid) pouching out (di/vert/ic/ul/um) from the small intestine. Although generally called "the appendix" its technical name is the "vermi/form (vermi- is a root also meaning "worm") (see Lesson 12 - appendic).

---

splanchn-, splanchno-   internal organs, viscera, entrails; heart, liver, intestines, etc.

Examples:
- splanchnectopia (splanchn/ec/top/ia)—out of place internal organ
- splanchnodynia (splanchn/odyn/ia)—pain in an internal organ
- eusplanchnia (eu/splanchn/ia)—a normal (good) condition of the internal organs

---

sta-, ste-, stas-   set, cause to stand, fix

This element carries meanings similar to those that we use in our words such as: sta/nd, sta/ble, sta/tionary, sta/tus, sta/ck, all of which carry the idea of remaining or being in a fixed position.

Example:
- stasis (sta/sis)—a stoppage of the flow of blood or other body fluid in any body part

-stasis (-sta/sis)—a stoppage, standing, arresting:
- diastasis (dia/sta/sis)—"standing apart"; a form of bone dislocation
- metastasis (meta/stasis)—"standing beyond"; the traveling of a disease process from one part of the body to another
- stasia (-stas/ia)—a condition of standing; a stoppage
  - cholestasia (chole/stas/ia)—stoppage or suppression of the flow of bile
- hemostasis, hemostasia (hem/o/sta/sis, hem/o/stas/ia)—the arrest of the escape of blood; the checking of the flow of blood
- hemostat (hem/o/stat)—anything used to stop bleeding; a clamplike instrument used in surgery; a medicine that hastens clotting

---

ton-   a stretching, tension

Example:
- tonometer (ton/o/meter)—an instrument to measure tension

The word ton/e, meaning a vocal or musical sound, originates in the noise produced by the vibrating of a stretched string. Vocal sounds are produced by the vibrating vocal cords under various stages of tens/ion or stretching. To be tens/e or under tens/ion is to be stretched, tight, strained, taut. To ex/tend is to stretch out producing an ex/tens/ion of greater or lesser ex/tent; to dis/tend is to stretch apart producing a dis/tens/ion. Here is a family of elements, all of which carry the idea of stretching:

tein- (tan-, ten-), tas-, tend-, tens- —to stretch, strain; tetan- —stretched; spasm:

- tone (ton/e)—the normal degree of vigor and tens/ion; in muscle, the resistance to stretching when in a relaxed state
- tonic (ton/ic)—producing and restoring the normal tone
- atony (a/ton/y)—"not tone"; lack of tone
- tentanus (tetan/us)—lockjaw; an acute infectious disease characterized by spasmodic contractions and rigidity of some or all of the voluntary muscles
- bronchotetany (bronch/o/tetan/y)—bronch/o/spasm; contraction of the bronchial tubes due to excessive constriction of the muscles surrounding them

-ectasy (-ec/tas/y)—a stretching; the act of stretching:

- lithectasy (lith/ec/tas/y)—removal of a stone through the stretched urethra

volv-   to turn, roll, roll over; a turning or rolling

volut- —a turning or rolling motion

Examples:

- volvulus (volv/ul/us)—intestinal obstruction due to a knotting and twisting of the bowel
- volvulate (volv/ul/ate)—to twist or form a knot

The prefix *volute-* denotes a rolling or turning motion. To re/volve is to turn back or turn again. A re/volut/ion is a rolling back of authority. To be in/volv/ed is to be rolled up in some occupation, cause or person. E/volut/ion is a "turning out," an "unfolding." The word "volume" comes from the ancient writings in the form of scrolls which were rolled up sheets of parchment.

Examples:

- convolution (con/volut/ion)—"rolled together"; a twisting, coiling or winding together; specifically, any of the folds or ridges on the surface of the brain
- involute (in/volut/e)—to return (re/turn) to normal size after enlargement
- subinvolution (sub/in/volut/ion)—"less than re/turn"; incomplete
- involution (in/volut/ion; failure of a part to return to its normal size and condition after enlargement

xer-   dry

Examples:
- xerosis (xer/osis)—abnormal dryness as of the eye or skin
- xeroderma (xer/o/derm/a)—"dry skin"; dryness and roughness of the skin
- xerocheilia (xer/o/cheil/ia)—"dry lips"; dryness of the lips

☞ **Note:** The original "Xerox" (Xer/ox) copier was so named because it was a dry copier. It was in total contrast to the wet copiers of the time that used photographic processes.

Lesson 14—Element Recognition

Separate the word terminals, elements, and connecting vowels of the following medical terms from right to left by inserting a slash mark (/) between them.

apogeny

blastoma

dimorphic

diameter

disable

eurycephalous

leptodermic

lymphadenoma

medial

metamorphosis

miocardia

monomorphous

necrectomy

pectus

pernasal

proximal

hemorrhage

diarrhea

scoliosis

splanchnodynia

hemostasis

tonic

volvulus

xerocheilia

Lesson 14—Interpretation Exercise

Complete the following statements by printing the meanings of the elements that make up the medical term in the proper blanks. (Remember, most medical terms are interpreted from right to left.)

14-1. The term apogeny (apo/gen/y) denotes the _____ of power to _____.

14-2. The term blastula (blast/u/la), which means _____ _____, is the name given to an embryo in its early stages.

14-3. The term dihysteria (di/hyster/ia) denotes having _____ _____.

14-4. Dialysis (dia/lysis), which means_____ _____, is a process by which substances are separated especially impurities from blood during kidney failure.

14-5. The term dissect (dis/sect) means to _____ _____.

14-6. Eurycephalous (eury/cephal/ous) denotes having a _____ _____.

14-7. Facial (faci/al) is a term pertaining to the _____.

14-8. The term leptodactyly (lept/o/dactyl/y) denotes abnormally _____ _____ and/or _____.

14-9. Lymphaden (lymph/aden) refers to a _____ _____.

14-10. The term mesonasal (mes/o/nasal) denotes being situated in the _____ of the _____.

14-11. Metaplasia (meta/plas/ia) is a term used to denote_____ _____ of one type of tissue to another.

14-12. Osteomiosis (oste/o/mio/sis) denotes a condition of _____ _____.

14-13. The term monomorphous (mono/morph/ous) refers to having a _____ _____.

14-14. A necrectomy (necr/ectomy) is the surgical_____ of _____ tissue.

14-15. Pectoralgia (pector/algia) denotes_____ in the _____.

14-16. The term percutaneous (per/cutan/eous) means _____ the _____.

14-17. The term proximal (proxim/al) pertains to being _____.

14-18. Enterorrhagia (enter/o/rrhag/ia) is a term that denotes _____ _____.

14-19. Diarrhea (dia/rrhe/a), which means to _____ _____, is used to signify an excessive looseness or frequency of bowel movement.

14-20. Scoliosis (scoli/osis) is a _____ of _____ associated mostly with the spine.

14-21. The term splanchnodynia (splanchn/odyn/ia) denotes _____ in an _____ _____.

14-22. A hemostat (hem/o/stat) is used to _____ the flow of_____.

14-23. A tonometer (ton/o/meter) is an instrument used to measure _____.

14-24. The term convolution (con/volut/ion) denotes being _____ _____.

14-25. The term xeroderma (xer/o/derm/a) denotes _____ _____.

Reference Section
and
Final Test

Familiar Elements

There are a number of useful medical elements imbedded in words with which you are familiar. The purpose of this section is to make you aware of these elements, to give them a medical definition, and to show you how they are related to medical terms.

---

abdomin-   the abdomen; the belly; the part of the body, except for the back, between the thorax (chest) and the pelvis (hip area)

Examples:
- abdominal (abdomin/al)—pertaining to the abdomen
- abdominous (abdomin/ous)—"full abdomen"; big-bellied
- abdominalgia (abdomin/algia)—"belly-ache"; pain in the abdomen
- abdominocardiac (abdomin/o/cardi/ac)—pertaining to the abdomen and the heart
- abdominohysterectomy (abdomin/o/hyster/ectomy)—hysterectomy performed through an abdominal incision; a hysterectomy performed through the abdomen (abdominal hysterectomy), as opposed to a hysterectomy performed through the vagina (vaginal hysterectomy)

---

ana-   up, up from below

To analyze is to "loosen up," to separate (a thing, idea, etc.) into its parts. Ana/tomy is a "cutting up," the dissecting of a plant or animal in order to examine its parts. Ana/tomy, therefore, has come to be known as the science of the form and structure of plants or animals based on the "cutting up" which has been performed:

- anastomosis (ana/stom/osis)—"a state of joining up by mouths or openings"; an interconnect in between blood vessels; a surgical procedure whereby one hollow or tubular organ is joined to another
- anaplastic (ana/plast/ic)—"forming back"; restoring a lost or missing part
- anaplasty (ana/plast/y)—restorative or plastic surgery

---

bio- (bi-)   life

You have seen this root in:
- biology (bio/logy)—"life science"; the science that deals with living matter
- biography (bio/graph/y)—"life writing"; written history of a person's life

Medical applications include:
- biopsy (bi/ops/y)—"appearance of life" (*ops-* look, appearance, view; related to *op-*, *ops-* "see"); the removal of tissues, cells, or fluids from the living body for examination or study

-bio/tic—pertaining to life:
- antibiotic (anti/bio/tic)—a substance produced by a microorganism (such as bacteria) having the capacity to inhibit the growth or kill another microorganism (such as a disease germ); in this sense, tending to inhibit or destroy life

brevi-   short

You have seen this root in:
- brevity (brevi/ty)—shortness of duration; shortness of time
- abbreviate (ab/brevi/ate)—to shorten; to make brief

Medical applications include:
- brevilingual (brevi/lingu/al)—"short tongued"
- breviflexor (brevi/flex/or)—a short flexor muscle

cav-, cavit-   hollow

This root is familiar in:
- cave (cav/e)—a hollow space inside the earth
- cavity (cavit/y)—a hole or hollow place; a hollow space in a tooth especially when caused by decay; a natural hollow place within the body
- cavern—a cave, especially a large cave

The root carries medical meanings:
- cav—a small enclosed space within the body or an organ
- cavit—appearing as "cavit/y"; used to designate hollow spaces in the body and lesions of a tooth produced by dental caries
- cavern—the general element used to designate a cavity

Examples:
- cavernoscopy (cavern/o/scop/y)—inspection of the cavities of the lung by means of an instrument
- concave (con/cave)—"very hollow"; hollow and curved like the inside half of a hollow ball
- cavernous (cavern/ous)—"full of caves"; containing caverns or hollow spaces

circum-   around

This prefix is familiar in:
- circumference (circum/ference)—the line forming the boundary of ("surrounding") a circle
- circumstantial (circum/stantial)—as in "circumstantial evidence" or in the phrase "depending on the circumstances." In both of these phrases the *circum-* root carries the meaning of "surrounding" or "around."

The same idea of "around," "about," "on all sides" applies to medical words:

- circumoral (circum/or/al)—around or near the mouth
- circumrenal (circum/ren/al)—around or near the kidney
- circumduction (circum/duct/ion)—"draw around"; the circular movement of a limb or of an eye

---

com-, con-   with, together, completely

To compress (com/press) is to press together. Concentric (con/centr/ic) circles are circles having the same center or having a center "together" with each other.

---

dist-   far

Familiar in:

- distant (dist/ant), distance (dist/ance), outdistance (out/dist/ance), all of which carry the meanings of "far," "away from"

Medical term:

- distal (dist/al)—remote; farther from any point of reference

---

EENT   ear, eye, nose, throat

This is an acronym (recall *acr-* meaning "tip, extremity" and *-nym* as in audi/o/nym meaning "name"). An acronym is a word formed from the first letters of a series of words; in this case (E)ar, (E)ye, (N)ose, (T)hroat. Although EENT is not a medical word, it is commonly used to designate the area of medical practice specializing in ear, eye, nose, and throat disease and conditions.

---

en-, em-   in, within, into (same as *in-*)

To enclose (en/close) is to close in. To embrace (em/brace) is to fold in, to hug.

---

fibr-   fiber, filament

A fiber is a slender threadlike structure. We recognize the word as it applies to textiles such as wool fibers, cotton fibers, nylon fibers, etc. Our bodies contain structures that are made up of similar long threadlike strands. Nerves and muscles are notable examples. Tumors may consist either partially or entirely of fibrous (fibr/ous) contents.

Examples:

- fibril (fibr/il)—a very small fiber
- fibroma (fibr/oma)—a tumor composed mainly of fibr/ous tissue
- lipofibroma (lip/o/fibr/oma)—a fibr/oma containing fatty elements
- fibromuscular (fibr/o/muscul/ar)—composed of fibr/ous and muscular tissue

flex-, flect-   to bend, turn

Did you ever flex your muscles? How many times have you seen your reflection (re/flect/ion) in a mirror? Bending was involved in both cases. In the case of the mirror light was reflected (re/flect/ed) or bent back toward your eyes.

Examples:
- flexure (flex/ure)—a bending; a bent portion of a structure or organ
- circumflex (circum/flex)—"bent around"; curved like a bow; a structure which has the form of a bent bow
- retroflexion (retro/flex/ion)—"bending backward"; the bending of an organ so that its top is turned backward; essentially, a U-shape.

in-   in, within; not

This prefix signifies the meanings "in," "into," or "within" as in:
- inpatient (in/patient)—a patient maintained and treated in the hospital
- inject (in/ject)—force into
- inside (in/side)—within the side, within

It is also used to convey the negative meaning of "not":
- inoperable (in/oper/able)—not operable
- inorganic (in/organ/ic)—not organic
- inactive (in/act/ive)—not active

In the usage of the prefix *"in-"* for the meaning "not," the letter "n" changes to the letter "l," "m," or "r" before words that begin with that same letter. Examples:
- illogical (il/log/ical)—not logical
- immovable (im/mov/able)—not movable
- irregular (ir/reg/ular)—not regular

infer-	below
infero-	below and_____; on the underside and_____
infra-	beneath

We can readily recognize the meanings "below" or "under" or "lower" in the words inferior (infer/ior) and inferiority (infer/ior/ity). In our ordinary usage the meaning is figurative in the sense that achievement, status, quality, etc., are lower than or under or below some acceptable standard. Inferior and inferiority are contrasted with superior (super/ior) and superiority (super/ior/ity).

In medical terms, *infer-* and *infero-* usually mean located underneath, below, on the under side of. In medical terminology we discussed the element *infra-* meaning "beneath." To summarize:

infer- almost always in the form "infer/ior," means "situated below" or "directed downward"; usually to refer to the lower surface of an organ or other structure.

infero—used with another word element as a directional pointer; below and . . . (See below, that is, the infer/ior part of this duscussion)

infra—used with another word element, also as a direction pointer meaning situated, formed, or occurring beneath

Examples:

- inferolateral (infero/later/al)—situated below and to one side
- inferomedian (infero/medi/an)—situated in the middle of the underside
- inferoposterior (infero/poster/ior)—situated below and behind
- infraumbilical (infra/umbilic/al)—beneath the navel or "belly button"

loc-   place

Local (loc/al) means "pertaining to a place." A location (loc/ation) is a place. To locate (loc/ate) means to find a place.

Examples:

- locus (loc/us)—a place
- loculus (loc/ul/us)—"a small place"; a small space or cavity
- loculi (loc/ul/i)—"small places"; plural of luc/ul/us
- dislocation (dis/loc/ation)—"apart from place"; the dis/place/ment of any part, more especially of a bone

mono-   one, alone, single; limited to one part

A monotone (mono-tone) is one tone or a single tone. Monogamy (mono/gamy) means being married to only one person. A monoplane (mono/plane) has a single wing.

Examples:

- monolayer (mono/layer)—consisting of a single layer
- monoplegia (mono/pleg/ia)—paralysis of a single part
- monosteotic (mon/oste/o/tic)—pertaining to or affecting a single bone

multi-   many, much; having or consisting of more than one

A multitude (multi/tude) is a large number of things or persons. To multiply (multi/ply) is to increase in number. Multicolored (multi/colored) is more than one color.

Examples:

- multiform (multi/form)—occurring in many forms
- multirooted (multi/rooted)—having more than one root as the molar teeth
- multi-articular—pertaining to or affecting many joints

muscul- muscle

We readily recognize a muscular (muscul/ar) person as one having well-developed or prominent muscles:

- musculocutaneous (muscul/o/cut/aneous)—pertaining to or supplying both muscles and skin
- intermuscular (inter/muscul/ar)—situated between muscles

narc, narcot- numbness, stupor, lethargy

We are very much aware of the problems caused by narcotics (narcot/ics) including the numbing effect which many of these substances produce. Narcosis (narc/osis) is the "condition of numbness" that can be produced by narcotics.

Examples:

- electronarcosis (electr/o/narc/osis)—electroshock; unconsciousness produced by passing an electric current through the brain of a patient; used in treating some forms of mental illness
- encephalonarcosis (en/cephal/o/narc/osis)—stupor due to brain disease
- narcotism (narcot/ism)—addiction to narcot/ics

nas- nose

This root is familiar in such expressions involving the nose as "nasal (nas/al) voice," "nasal spray," "nasal drip."

Examples:

- pernasal (per/nas/al)—"through the nose"; performed through the nose, such as a surgical procedure or injection
- nasopharynx (nas/o/pharynx)—the space where the nasal passages enter the pharynx
- subnasal (sub/nasal)—situated below the nose

nox, nos- disease, illness

A noxious (nox/ious) gas is one which can cause illness. An obnoxious (ob/nox/ious) person is one who is so unpleasant or offensive as to figuratively be "sickening."

-nosis (-nos/is)—word ending indicating disease:

- trophonosis (troph/o/nos/is)—any disease or disorder due to nutritional causes
- trichonosis (trich/o/nos/is)—any disease of the hair
- hematonosis (hemat/o/nos/is)—any disease of the blood

-nosology (-nos/ology)—word ending denoting the classification of diseases:

- nosology (nos/ology)—the science of the classification of diseases
- dermonosology (derm/o/nos/ology)—the classification of skin diseases
- nosogenic (nos/o/gen/ic)—causing disease

---

palat-   palate; the roof of the mouth consisting of a hard bony forward part (the hard palate) and a soft fleshy back part (the soft palate)

This root is familiar in the word "palatable" (palat/able) by which we mean pleasant or acceptable to the taste. We now know that the sense of taste (taste buds) is principally in the tongue. However the earlier idea that taste arose from the roof of the mouth (the palate) persists in the word "palatable."

Examples:

- palatoglossal (palat/o/gloss/al)—pertaining to the roof of the mouth (palate) and tongue
- transpalatal (trans/palat/al)—performed through the roof of the mouth
- palatoplasty (palat/o/plasty)—plastic reconstruction of the palate, including cleft palate operations
- cleft palate (cleft palat/e)—a con/genit/al deformity consisting of a fiss/ure (cleft) from front to back along the middle of the mouth

---

pelvi-, pelv-, pelvis   the basin-like cavity formed by the ring of bones in the lower back part of the trunk, supporting the spinal column and resting on the legs

Most of us, having seen human skeletons or their representations, and being aware of the bony structure of our own bodies, know that the pelvis is somewhere in the area of our hips. For the purpose of applying medical terminology we need to know that it consists of the ring of bones forming a basin like structure in the area where our spinal column ends and from which our thigh bones extend.

Examples:

- intrapelvic (intra/pelv/ic)—within the pelvis
- pelvimeter (pelvi/meter)—an instrument for measuring the diameters and space (capacity) of the pelvis

---

proxim-   near

We encounter *proxim-* in: proximity (proxim/ity), as in the sentence, "The disturbance occurred in the proximity of (near) City Hall."

approximate (ap/proxim/ate) or approximately (ap/proxim/ate/ly), as in, "It takes approximately (nearly) three hours to go from here to there."

Medical term:

- proximal (proxim/al)—nearest; closer to any point of reference

In medical descriptions major points of reference are:

the center of the body; an imaginary line drawn from the middle of the forehead and continuing to the space between the two feet, thus dividing the body into two halves

points of attachment such as the shoulder by which the arm is connected with the main part (or trunk) of the body

re-   back, back again; contrary, opposite

The prefix *re-* appears in many words we commonly use: readmit (re/admit), reaffirm (re/affirm), reappear (re/appear), reassemble (re/assemble), reassign (re/assign), reawaken (re/awaken), reattempt (re/attempt), reauthorize (re/authorize). Note that we have attached *re-* to a few words at the beginning of the alphabet. There are many more words which can be formed using *re-* as a prefix.

Examples:

- reaction (re/action)—opposite action, or counteraction
- reflex (re/flex)—"bend back"; "bend again"; a kind of "re/action"
- reflex action (re/flex action)—an "automatic" response as in unthinkingly raising a hand to ward off a blow
- respiration (re/spir/ation)—"breathing back"; the "back and forth" action of the lungs in inhalation and exhalation

sect- (-sect)   a cut or division; to cut or divide

To dissect (dis/sect) is to cut apart; to bisect (bi/sect) is to cut in two; to intersect (inter/sect) is to cut between; a section (sect/ion) is a division or "cutting out"; a religious sect is one which has broken away ("cut out" or split away) from an established church.

In medical terminology the meaning is practically synonymous with *-otomy* in designating the act, process, or product of cutting; specifically, an incision in surgery.

Examples:

- trans section (trans/sect/ion)—"cut across"; the process of cutting across or dividing by cutting
- resection (re/sect/ion)—"cut again" (in the sense of being recut or cut out); the surgical removal of part of an organ, bone, etc. Compare *-ectomy*, "surgical removal," with re/sect/ion, "surgical removal of part of."
- cesarean sect/ion—incision through the abdominal and uterine walls for the delivery of a fetus

skelet, skeleton   the bony framework of the body

The element *skelet-* fairly leaps out at us from the familiar words skeletal (skelet/al) and skeleton (skelet/on).

Examples:
- skeletal (skelet/al)—pertaining to the bones of the body
- skeletal (skelet/al) system—the bones of the body acting together in their functions to provide support and give shape to the body, and, with the attached tendons, muscles, and ligaments, make body movement possible.
- endoskeletal (end/o/skelet/al)—pertaining to the bones of the body enclosed by the skin and muscles, as distinguished from exo/skelet/al
- exoskeletal (exo/skeletal)—pertaining to a hard structure developed on the outside of the body such as the shell of a crab or turtle; also applied to the hard outer structures in humans such as hair, nails, or teeth.

super-   over, over and above (in the sense of excessive); higher in quantity, quality, or degree

Examples:
- supercilium (super/cili/um)—"over the eyelid or eyelash"; the eyebrow
- superlethal (super/lethal)—"excessively lethal"; more than enough to cause death
- supercerebral (super/cerebr/al)—in the upper part of the cerebrum

tors-, tort-   twist, turn

A contortionist (con/tort/ion/ist) is a person, usually a theatrical or circus acrobat, who can twist his body into unnatural positions. Torture (tort/ure) comes from the twisting devices used to inflict severe pain. A tortuous (tort/uous) road is full of twists, turns, curves, and windings. To distort (dis/tort) may be to literally twist some object out of shape or, figuratively, to twist a fact or facts.

Examples:
- detorsion (de/tors/ion)—the correction of a curvature or deformity
- torticollis (tort/i/coll/is)—"twisted neck" (*coll-* 'neck'); wry neck; a spasm or contraction of the muscles on one side of the neck, causing the head to be tilted and twisted

tox-   poison

You may know that a toxic (tox/ic) substance is a substance that is poisonous. Although intoxication (in/tox/ic/ation) is usually associated with an excessive use of alcohol, in medicine the word means poisoning or becoming poisoned by any substance such as alcohol and other drugs, serums, acids, etc.

Examples:

- toxin (tox/in)—a poison; a poisonous substance usually released by bacteria
- antitoxin (anti/toxin)—"against poison"; a neutralizer of a toxin; antibody (a counter poison) produced in the body which is capable of producing a specific immunity to a specific germ or virus
- toxemia (tox/em/ia)—condition resulting from poisons circulating in the blood
- ectotoxemia (ecto/tox/em/ia)—toxemia produced by a substance introduced from outside the body

ultra- beyond, excessive

To be ultraconservative (ultra/conservative) is to be excessively conservative. To be ultramodern (ultra/modern) is to be modern beyond the current norm. Ultrasonic (ultra/sonic) designates a frequency of mechanical vibrations beyond the range our ears can hear.

Examples:

- ultraligation (ultra/lig/ation)—ligation (tying) of a vessel beyond the point of origin of a branch
- ultrasome (ultra/some)—any body so small that it is invisible (beyond seeing) even when aided by the most powerful microscope
- ultravirus (ultra/virus)—an extremely (excessively) small disease-producing agent

vertebr-, vertebra any of the single bones or segments of the spinal column

Here is another element which seems obvious. A vertebra or the plural vertebrae is well known from courses in biology or health that we have taken. See *spondyl-* in Reading Assignment of Lesson 4.

Examples:

- vertebrate (vertebr/ate)—having a spinal column or backbone; any of the animals including all mammals, fishes, birds, reptiles, and amphibians which have a spinal column
- invertebrate (in/vertebr/ate)—"not vertebr/ate"; lacking a spinal column; a division of the animal kingdom which includes all animals other than mammals, fishes, birds, reptiles, and amphibians
- vertebrarterial (vertebr/arteri/al)—pertaining to the vertebr/al artery (an artery carrying blood to the vertebrae)

Application of Elements to Medical Classifications

Branches of Medicine

ana/tomy	"cut up"; science of the structure of the body and relationship of its parts
embry/ology	"study of the first stages of the fertilized egg"; study of the formation and development of the embryo
hist/ology	"study of tissue"; study of the structure, composition, and function of normal cells and tissues
path/ology	"study of disease"; study of the changes in the structure or functions of the body caused by disease
physi/ology	"study of the body"; study of the normal functions and activities of the body

Major Medical Specialties and Specialists

Two endings dominate the words designating medical specialties: -*ology* which in this application means, broadly, "study of" and, more narrowly, "science of"; -*iatry* or -*iatrics*: carries the meaning "healing" or "treatment of disease."

There are corresponding endings used to form the words designating the specialist, the "one who," the "healer": -*ist* generally combines with -*olog(y)* to form -*olog/ist*, and -*iatr(y)* to form -*iatrist*; -*ian* combines with -*iatric(s)* to form -*iatrician*.

an/esthes/i/ology	"science of lack of feeling"; dealing with the administration of an/esthet/ic/s to produce loss of feeling or consciousness, usually in conjunction with forms of medical treatment such as surgery *an/esthes/i/ologist - the specialist*
cardi/ology	"science of the heart"; dealing with the heart and its diseases *cardi/ologist - the specialist*
dermat/ology	"science of the skin"; dealing with the skin and its diseases *dermat/ologist - the specialist*
ear, eye, nose, throat	frequently referred to as EENT or ENT for ear, nose, and throat only
end/o/crin/ology	"science of secreting within"; dealing with the end/o/crin/e glands and their internal secretions (products of the thyroid, parathyroids, adrenals, pancreas, testicles, ovaries, pituitary, pineal, thymus, and testes) *end/o/crin/ologist - the specialist*
ger/i/atrics	"treatment of disease of old age"; dealing with the diseases and hygiene of old age *ger/iatrician - the specialist*

Major Medical Specialties and Specialists (cont.)

gynec/ology	"science of females"; dealing with the specific functions and diseases of women *gynec/ologist - the specialist*
internal medicine	science dealing with the diagnosis and nonsurgical treatment of disease *intern/ist - the specialist (note: not to be confused with the word "intern", an "intern" is a recent medical school graduate serving an apprenticeship in a hospital)*
laryng/ology	"science of throat"; dealing with the throat and its diseases *laryng/ologist - the specialist*
neur/ology	"science of the nerves"; dealing with the nervous system and its diseases *neur/ologist - the specialist*
obstetr/ics	originally derived from a term applied to a midwife literally meaning "she who stands before" (*ob-* before and *stetr-*, a variation of *sta-* to stand); dealing with the care and treatment of women during pregnancy, childbirth, and the period immediately following *obstetr/ician - the specialist*
onc/ology	"science of tumors"; dealing with the study and treatment of tumors *onc/ologist - the specialist*
ophthalm/ology	"science of the eye"; dealing with the structure, functions, and diseases of the eye *ophthalm/ologist - the specialist*
orth/o/ped/ics (orth/o/ped/ic surgery)	"child straightening"; surgery dealing with the treatment of deformities diseases, and injuries of bones, joints, muscles, ligaments, etc. So called because many deformities are con/genit/al and as such are discovered and corrected in childhood *orth/o/ped/ist - the specialist (may also be called "orth/o/ped/ic surgeon" or, more briefly, "orthopod.")*
ot/ology	"science of the ear"; dealing with the structure, function, and diseases of the ear *ot/ologist - the specialist*
ped/iatrics	"science of the child"; dealing with the hygienic care and diseases of children *ped/iatrician - the specialist*
plast/ic surgery	"reparative surgery"; surgery dealing with the repair or restoration of injured, deformed, or destroyed parts of the body, especially by transferring tissue, such as skin or bone, from other parts of the ones own body or from that of another *plast/ic surgeon - the specialist*
proct/ology	"science of the rectum"; dealing with the rectum and anus and their diseases *proct/ologist - the specialist*

Major Medical Specialties and Specialists (cont.)

psych/iatry	"science of the mind"; concerned with the study, treatment, and prevention of disorders of the mind *psych/iatrist - the specialist*
pulmon/ology	"science of the lung"; dealing with the lungs and their diseases *pulmon/ologist - the specialist*
radi/ology	"science of rays"; dealing with X-rays and other forms of radiant energy X-raying body parts and treating diseases *radi/ologist - the specialist*
rhin/ology	"science of the nose"; dealing with the nose and its diseases *rhin/ologist - the specialist*
ur/ology	"science of the urinary tract"; dealing with the ur/o/genit/al or ur/in/ary system and its diseases *ur/ologist - the specialist*

Topographic Systems

The word topographic means "pertaining to description of place." The word system means "a placing together." Topographic systems are groupings of interconnected or interdependent organs which together accomplish some specific function in which these systems form the major categories within which diseases and operations are classified for record keeping and other display and reference usage.

body as a whole	includes the mind (psyche) and other regions that are a particular system exclusively
cardi/o/vas/cul/ar	"pertaining to the heart and vessels"; the heart and the blood vessels
digestive	the alimentary tract or canal; the tube beginning at the mouth and ending at the anus through which food is ingested, digested, and eliminated; includes the teeth, tongue, salivary glands, liver, and pancreas
end/o/crine	"secreting within"; the system of ductless glands including the thyroid, parathyroid, thymus, pituitary, pineal, adrenals
hem/ic and lymphat/ic	"pertaining to the blood and lymph"; the blood, lymph, spleen
in/tegument/ary	"pertaining to the covering (skin)"; the skin (including mucous membranes, glands of the skin, hair, nails, breast)
muscul/o/skelet/al	"pertaining to the muscles and bony framework"; the bones, muscles, joints, cartilages, bursas, ligaments, tendons

Topographic Systems (cont.)

nerv/ous   the nerves including the brain and spinal cord

organs of special   principally sight and hearing (eyes and ears)
sense

re/spirat/ory   "pertaining to breathing"; the nose, sinuses, larynx (voice box), trachea
                                  (windpipe), bronchial structures, lung, lung covering and chest cavity
                                  lining (pleura)

ur/o/genit/al   "pertaining to the urinary and genital"; kidney, bladder, urethra, internal
                                  and external reproductive organs, female genital organs during preg-
                                  nancy including the fetus and fetal structures

Medical Terms Used in the Description of Diseases

a/chlor/hydr/ia	see chlor/hydr/ia
a/chyl/la	(a- not + chyl- gastric juice) "not gastric juice"; partial or complete loss of gastric juice
a/gen/e/sis	(a- not + genesis- development) "not developed"; faulty or incomplete development
a/nom/aly	(a- not + nomaly- distributed) "not distributed"; not in a normal or expected position
a/plas/ia	(a- not + plasia- formation, development) "not formed"; the incomplete or faulty formation of an organ or part
a/spir/ation	(a- from ad- to + spiration- breathing) "to breathe"; the act of breathing or drawing in; also the removal of fluids or gases from a cavity by suction
a/tres/ia	(a- not + tres- hole or opening) "not opening"; absence or closure of a natural passage of the body
a/troph/y	(a- not + trophy- nourishment) "not nourished"; a wasting away or decrease in size as from disuse, old age, injury or disease
abs/cess	(ab- from abs- away + cess- go) Literally "to go away"; a localized collection of pus surrounded by inflamed tissue
ad/hes/ion	(ad- to + hesion- a sticking) "sticking to"; the abnormal union of surfaces normally separated by the formation of new fibrous tissue; also the union of the edges of a wound
aden/o/carcin/oma	(aden- gland + carcin- cancer + oma- tumor) "cancerous gland tumor"; a cancerous (malignant) tumor originating in glandular tissues such as the breast
aden/o/lymph/oma	(aden- gland + lymph + oma- tumor) "tumor of the lymph gland"; an adenoma (benign tumor of gland-like structure) of a lymph organ
aden/o/my/oma	(aden- gland + my- muscle + oma- tumor) "tumor of gland and muscle"; a benign tumor composed of muscular and glandular elements
aden/o/my/osis	(aden- gland + my- muscle + osis- condition) "condition of muscle and gland"; the presence of endometrial (lining of the uterus) material in the myometrium (muscular layer of the wall of the uterus); also called internal endometriosis
aden/oma	(aden- gland + oma- tumor) "tumor of gland"; a benign tumor of a gland-like structure
aero/phag/ia	(aer- air + phag- eat, swallow) "air swallowing"; the swallowing of air especially in hysteria
ag/glut/in/ation	(ag- from ad- to + glut- glue) "stick to"; the process of union in the healing of a wound; also, a reaction in which particles such as red blood cells, bacteria, and virus particles tend to cluster together when suspended in a liquid

amel/o/blast/oma	(amel- enamel + blast- bud + oma- tumor) "tumor of enamel buds or germ cells"; a tumor of the jaw formed from remnants of tooth enamel germ (bud or sprout) cells
amyl/oid	(amyl- starch + oid- resembling) "resembling starch, starchlike"; a starchlike substance; starchy food
an/orex/ia	(an- not, lacking + orexia- desire, appetite) "lacking appetite"; pathological loss of appetite from psychic causes frequently resulting from starvation diets
ana/plast/ic	(ana- back again + plast- to form) "form back again"; characterized by reversed development
angul/ation	(angul- angle) "process or connected with an angle"; an abnormal bend or curve in an organ
bi/furc/ation	(bi- two + furc- fork) "two-forked"; branching into two parts; division into two branches
bulim/ia	(bul- cattle + lim- hunger) "literally, hungry as cattle"; an abnormal and constant craving for food
calcar/eous	(calcar- of lime) "full of lime"; containing calcium or any calcium compound
calc/ul/us	(calc- stone + ul- small) "a small stone"; solid stonelike matter composed mostly of mineral salts, found mainly in hollow organs, ducts, passages, and cysts
carcin/oma	(carcin- cancer + oma- tumor) "cancerous tumor"; a malignant tumor
cardi/algia	(cardi- heart + algia- pain) "heart pain"; heartburn; pain in the heart
caud/al/ly	(caud- tail) "toward the tail"; in a direction more toward the tail or the rear hind part of the trunk
chlor/hydr/ia	(chlor- chlorine + hydr- water) a combination meaning "hydrochloric acid" or, more specifically, "hydrochloric acid in the gastric juice," essential in breaking food down into simpler chemical compounds which can be absorbed and used by the body
a/chlorhydria	(a- not + chlorhydria) "not hydrochloric acid"; absence of hydrochloric acid from the gastric juice
hyper/chlorhydria	(hyper- above, excessive + chlorhydria) "excessive hydrochloric acid"; the presence of a greater than typical proportion of hydrochloric acid in the gastric juice, especially characteristic of various pathological states such as ulceration
hypo/chlorhydria	(hypo- below, deficient + chlorhydria) "deficient hydrochloric acid"; deficiency of hydrochloric acid in the gastric juice
chol/angi/oma	(chole- bile + angi- vessel, duct + oma- tumor) "tumor of bile duct"; a tumor of the bile ducts
chondr/oma	(chondr- cartilage + oma- tumor) "tumor of cartilage"; a tumor composed of cartilage tissue
con/cret/ion	(con- together + cret- grow) "grow together"; a hard mass formed in a body cavity or in tissue
con/stip/ation	(con- together + stip- press) "press together"; abnormally delayed or infrequent movement of dry hardened feces

con/tract/ure   (con- together + tract- draw) "draw together"; deformity or distortion produced by scar tissue or a permanent shortening of muscles, tendons, or fascia

cyst   (cyst- pouch, bladder) "pouch"; a pouch lacking an opening but having a membrane and developing in a natural cavity of the body, in the substance of an organ, or in an abnormal structure such as a tumor; also a bladder, especially applied to the urinary and gall bladders

di/lat/ation   (di- from dis- apart + lat- wide) "wide apart"; the condition of being stretched beyond normal dimensions especially as a result of overwork or disease

di/vert/ic/ul/ation   (di from de- away from + vert- turn) "a turning away from"; the formation of abnormal pouches or sacs opening from a hollow organ such as the intestine or bladder

dia/rrhea   (dia- through + rrhe- flow) "flow through"; an abnormal frequency of discharge of more or less fluid waste products from the bowels

dis/loc/ation   (dis- apart + loc- place) "apart from place"; displacement of one or more bones at a joint; compare displacement, ectopia

dis/place/ment   (dis- apart + place-) "apart from place"; ectopia (out of place); removal from normal position or place; generally applied to other than out-of-position bones (dislocation) such as mental substitutes for reality, an out-of-place condition of the stomach, tissue change of position as a result of the pressure; compare dislocation, ectopia

dis/tort/ion   (dis- apart + tort- twist) "twisting apart"; the state of being twisted out of a natural or normal state or position

dors/al/ly   (dors- back) "backwardly"; in a back position or direction

duplic/ation   (duplic- double, twofold) "doubling"; the action or process of doubling especially applied to abnormal doublings or duplications in fetal development

dys/phag/ia   (dys- bad, difficult + phag- swallowing) "difficult swallowing"; difficulty in swallowing due to disease or accident

dys/plas/ia   (dys- bad, abnormal + plasia- development, growth) "abnormal development"; abnormal growth or development as of organs, tissues or cells

ef/fer/ent   (ef- from, ex- from, away from + fer- carry) "carry away from"; bearing or conducting outward from a part or organ; specifically, the conveying of nervous impulses from a center

e/long/ation   (e- from ex- from, away from + long- far, distant) "far away from"; the process or condition of increasing in length

e/ruct/ation   (e- from ex- from, forth + ruct- belch) "belch forth"; the act of belching gas from the stomach

ec/top/ia   (e from ex- from, away from + top- place) "away from place"; an abnormal congenital or acquired position of an organ or part such as the heart, crystalline lens, testicle, bladder; compare dislocation, displacement

em/bol/ism   (em- from in- in + bol- throw) "thrown in, stopped"; the sudden blocking of an artery by a clot or obstruction carried by the blood stream

em/bol/us   (em- from in- in + bol- throw) "throw in, stopper"; the clot or plug obstructing the blood flow in a blood vessel

end/arter/itis	(end- within + arter- artery + itis- inflammation) "inflammation within artery"; inflammation of the innermost lining of an artery
epi/derm/oid	(epi- above + derm- skin + oid- resembling) "resembling upper skin"; resembling the top skin layer (epidermis); composed of elements like those of the epidermis
epi/gastr/ium	(epi- above, over + gastr- stomach) "over the stomach"; the upper middle region of the abdomen
ex/trus/ion	(ex- from, out + trus- push, thrust) "push out"; a forcing out or expulsion; the condition of a tooth which extends above the bite line of the surrounding teeth
extra/vas/ation	(extra- outside, beyond + vas- vessel) "outside a vessel"; discharge or escape, as of blood into the tissues
fibr/o/sarc/oma	(fibr- fiber + sarc- flesh + oma- tumor) "tumor of fiber and flesh"; a tumor composed of fleshy and fibrous elements
fibr/oma	(fibr- fiber + oma- tumor) "fibrous tumor"; a tumor composed mainly of fibrous elements
fibr/osis	(fibr- fiber + osis- condition) "fibrous condition"; the formation of fibrous tissue; the degeneration of fibrous structures
fist/ul/a	(fistul- pipe) "pipe or passage"; an abnormal passage from an abscess, cavity, or hollow organ to the skin or to another abscess, cavity, or hollow organ
flacc/id	(flacc- flabby) "flabby"; weak, soft, lax; lacking tone, resilience, or firmness, especially muscles
fus/ion	(fus- melt) "union as if by melting"; the abnormal coherence of adjacent parts or bodies
gangli/o/neur/oma	(gangli- knot, swelling + neur- nerv + oma- tumor) "knotty nerve tumor"; a tumor growing from a nerve cell composed mainly of ganglion material; a tumor consisting of nerve and ganglion tissues
gangren/e	(gangren- gnawing away, an eating sore) "an eating away"; death of tissue, usually resulting from loss of blood supply
gli/osis	(gli- glue + osis- condition) "gluelike condition"; disease associated with excessive development of the supporting structure of nerve tissue
gran/ul/o/cyt/ic	(granul- little grain + cyt- cell) "pertaining to cells of small grainlike construction"; pertaining to a cell composed of grainlike particles
gran/ul/oma	(granul- little grain, little particle + oma- tumor) "grainy tumor"; a tumor or neoplasm made up of grainlike (granulation) tissue; a mass of chronically inflamed tissue marked by the formation of granulations
halit/osis	(halit- breath + osis- condition) "breath condition"; bad breath; offensive breath
hem/angi/oma	(hem- blood + angi- vessel + oma- tumor) "blood vessel tumor"; a usually benign tumor made up of blood vessels
hem/o/glob/in	(hem- blood + glob from globul- tiny ball) "tiny blood ball"; the red coloring matter of the red blood corpuscles serving to carry oxygen from the lungs to the tissues and carbon dioxide from the tissues to the lungs

hepat/o/megal/y	(hepat- liver + megaly- enlarged) "enlarged liver"; enlargement of the liver
hern/ia	(hern- intestine, entrails) "entrails condition"; rupture; the protrusion of all or part of an organ through a tear in the wall of the surrounding structure, especially the protrusion of the intestine through the abdominal muscles
hydr/o/peri/ton/eum	(hydr- water, fluid + peri- around + ton- stretch, stretched) "fluid in the stretched around"; note the peritoneum is the membrane that lines (stretched around) the abdominal cavity; ascites; abnormal accumulation of fluid in the abdominal cavity
hyper/chlor/hydr/ia	see chlorhydria
hyper/motil/ity	(hyper- above, excessive + motil- movement) "excessive movement"; abnormal or excessive movement; specifically, movement (motility) of all or part of the gastrointestinal tract; compare hypomotility
hyper/plas/ia	(hyper- above, excessive + plasia- formation) "excessive formation"; an abnormal or unusual increase in the elements composing a part such as the cells of a tissue
hyper/secret/ion	(hyper- above, excessive + secret- set apart) "excessive setting apart or separation"; excessive segregating or releasing of some material to perform a function (salivation) or for excretion (urination)
hyper/troph/y	(hyper- above, more than normal + trophy- nourishment, growth) "more than normal growth"; a considerable increase in the size of an organ or tissue
hypo/chlor/hydr/ia	see chlorhydria
hypo/motil/ity	(hypo- below, deficient + motil- movement) "deficient movement"; abnormal or diminished movement; specifically movement (motility) of body parts and functions; compare hypermotility
im/pact/ion	(im- from in- within, together + pact- press) "press together"; the condition of being firmly lodged (packed); specifically, of teeth which are so imbedded as to prevent eruption, or hardened feces in the rectum
in/carcer/ation	(in- in, within + carcer- prison) "imprisonment"; constricted, abnormal retention or confinement of a body part; specifically the constriction of the neck of a hernial sac
in/clus/ion	(in- in + clus- close) "closed or shut in"; anything that is enclosed; specifically, a lifeless constituent of a cell, or a tooth so surrounded with bony material that it is unable to erupt
in/continence	(in- not, lack + contin- hold, contain) "not holding"; lacking control; unrestrained; especially, uncontrolled sexual desire or inability to contain a bodily discharge such as urine
in/volut/ion	(in- in, inner + volut- rolling) "an inner rolling or rolling within"; a shrinking such as the return of the uterus to its former size after delivery, or the shriveling of an organ in an aged person, or the decrease in bodily vigor in women during menopause
leio/my/o/sarc/oma	(leio- smooth + my- muscle + sarc- flesh + oma- tumor) "smooth, muscle, fleshy tumor"; a fleshy tumor containing smooth muscle elements
les/ion	(les- injure, hurt) "an injury"; injury; impairment; flaw; an abnormal change or loss of function in a part or organ due to injury or disease

lig/ation	(lig- tie, bind) "tied or bound"; something that binds; also the surgical act of binding or tying
lip/o/sarc/oma	(lip- fat + sarc- flesh + oma- tumor) "fat, fleshy tumor"; a fleshy tumor containing fatty elements
lip/oma	(lip- fat + oma- tumor) "fatty tumor"; a tumor made up of fat cells
lymph/angi/oma	(lymph- watery fluid, lymph + angi- vessel + oma- tumor) "lymph vessel tumor"; a tumor formed of lymphatic vessels
lymph/o/sarc/oma	(lymph- watery fluid, lymph + sarc- flesh + oma- tumor) "lymph, fleshy tumor"; a general term applied to malignant neoplastic disorders of lympoid tissue, particularly a malignant tumor which spreads (metastisizes) to adjacent glands
lymph/oid	(lymph- watery fluid, lymph + oid- resembling) "resembling lymph, lymph-like"; resembling the tissue characteristics of lymph glands
malign/ancy	(mal- bad, evil, or malign- acting evilly) "bad action, evil action", a cancerous tumor; exhibiting cancerous qualities
medull/ary	(medull- marrow, pith) "of the pith or inner substance"; resembling marrow; pertaining to the innermost part (pith) of an organ or structure
melan/oma	(melan- black + oma- tumor) "black tumor"; a tumor made up of black-pigmented cells
melan/osis	(melan- black + osis- condition) "black condition"; a condition characterized by deposits of black or other pigmentary deposits in the tissues of the body
mes/o/thel/i/oma	(mes- middle + thel- nipple, cellular tissue + oma- tumor) "middle cellular tissue tumor"; a tumor derived from tissue such as that lining the peritoneum or pleura (mesothelial)
meta/bol/ism	(meta- beyond, change + bol- throw, thrust) "thrust beyond"; the chemical and physical processes (changes) continuously going on in the body and its constituent parts; the bodily processes of assmiliating food and breaking food down into simpler substances to provide repairs and energy
meta/sta/tic	(meta- beyond, change + sta- stand, place) "pertaining to placing beyond, spreading"; pertaining to the spread of disease from one part of the body to another
my/o/blast/oma	(my- muscle + blast- bud, sprout + oma- tumor) "muscle bud tumor"; a tumor in the muscle made up of groups of cells which resemble primitive (sprout) muscle cells
myel/oma	(myel- marrow, spinal cord + oma- tumor) "bone marrow tumor"; a tumor of the bone marrow
necr/osis	(necr- dead + osis- condition) "dead condition"; death of living tissue as may be caused by loss of blood supply, burning, local lesion of a disease, or injury
neo/plas/m	(neo- new + plas- growth) "a new growth"; any new or abnormal growth such as a tumor; may be benign, potentially malignant, or malignant
neur/o/fibr/oma	(neur- nerv + fibr- fiber + oma- tumor) "nerve and fiber tumor"; a fibrous tumor originating in the fibrous tissue of a nerve sheath

non/fus/ion	(non- not, lack + fus- melt, join) "lack of joining"; failure of parts, such as the edges of a wound, to properly join
ob/stip/ation	(ob- completely, totally + stip- press) "pressing completely or totally"; severe and persistent constipation
oc/clus/ion	(oc- from ob- completely, totally + clus- close) "close completely"; shutting off or obstruction of something such as the obstruction of the flow of blood to the heart (coronary occlusion); a closing or shutting such as the meeting of the teeth when the jaws are closed
opac/ity	(opac- dark, shaded) "condition of darkness"; darkness; a dark (opaque) spot on a normally transparent structure such as the cornea or lens of the eye
oste/oma	(oste- bone + oma- tumor) "bone tumor"; a tumor composed of bone tissue
papill/ary	(papill- nipple) "nipple-like"; pertaining to a nipple or resembling a nipple such as the small protuberances on the upper surface of the tongue
papill/oma	(papill- nipple + oma- tumor) "nipple-like tumor"; a benign tumor such as a wart or pimple growing on the surface of the skin (epithelium)
par/en/chym/atous	(par from para- beside, alongside + en from in- in + chym from chein- to pour) "relating to pour in beside (from the belief that the tissue of internal organs was poured in by the blood vessels)"; the essential elements of an organ (as a gland) or an abnormal growth (as a tumor) as distinguished from its supporting framework
par/esis	(par- from para- beside, at the side + esis- let go, send) "action of letting go, letting fall at the side"; slight or partial paralysis
para/sym/path/etic	(para- beyond, beside + sym- with + path- feeling) "feeling with beside or beyond"; properly the parasympathetic nervous system; the part of the nervous system whose functions include the constriction of the pupils of the eyes, the slowing of the heartbeat, and the stimulation of certain digestive glands
path/o/gen/ic	(path- feeling, suffering, disease + gen- producing, originating) "production of suffering or disease"; pertaining to the production or development of disease
peri/ton/eal	(peri- around, surrounding + ton- stretch) "stretched around"; pertaining to the membrane lining the abdominal cavity
petechiae	(petechiae, small spots produced in some infectious diseases) "contagious disease spot"; small, pinpoint, nonraised, perfectly round, purplish red spots appearing on the skin in some contagious diseases such as typhoid fever
pica	(pica- magpie, a bird that eats everything) "as non-discriminating as a magpie"; a craving for unnatural articles of food brought on by nutritional deficiencies or occurring in insanity; also, sometimes exhibited during pregnancy
plasm/a	(plasm- something formed) "formation"; the fluid part of the blood, lymph, milk, or intramuscular liquid, especially the fluid part of the blood (as distinguished from the corpuscles) used for transfusions
plate/let/s	(plate- from platy- broad, flat + let- little) "little plates"; a tiny flattened body, especially any of the small disks containing no hemoglobin, found in the blood and associated with the process of blood clotting

poly/dips/ia	(poly- many, much + dips- thirst) "much thirst"; excessive or abnormal thirst
poly/p	(poly- many + p shortened from pous- from pod- foot) "many feet"; a protruding growth from any mucous membrane, especially the mucous membrane of the nose. (the "many feet" applies to the roots of the growth)
pre/malign/ant	(pre- before + malign- cancerous) "before malignancy"; preceeding the development of malignancy; precancerous
pro/lap/se	(pro- before, forward + lapse- falling) "falling forward"; the falling or slipping out of place of an internal organ
pro/trus/ion	(pro- before, forth + trusion- thrusting) "thrusting forth"; a thrusting or jutting out
proct/algia	(proct- rectum + algia- pain) "pain in the rectum"; pain in the rectum
prol/i/fer/ation	(prol- offspring + fer- bear, carry) "bearing offspring"; multiply rapidly; the reproduction or multiplication of similar forms, especially of cells and morbid cysts
pt/osis	(pt- fall + osis- condition) "falling condition"; a prolapse; the falling of some organ or part, especially the drooping of the upper eyelid, caused by the paralysis of its muscle
ptyal/ism	(ptyal- saliva) "action pertaining to spit"; excessive secretion of saliva
pyl/or/ic	(pylor- gatekeeper) "pertaining to gatekeeping"; pertaining to the opening (gate) from the stomach into the first part of the small intestine (the pylorus)
rupt/ure	(rupt- break) "act of breaking"; breaking apart; bursting; a forcible tearing or bursting of an organ or part, as of a blood vessel, the bladder, etc.
scirrh/ous	(scirrh- hard) "resembling hardness"; resembling a hard cancerous tumor
scler/osis	(scler- hard + osis- condition) "hard condition"; a pathological hardening of tissue as in arteriosclerosis, multiple sclerosis
sen/ile	(sen- old) "having to do with age"; typical of or resulting from old age, especially the mental impairment characterized by confusion, memory loss, etc.
sin/us	(sin- curve, fold) "a fold"; any of various cavities, hollows and passages, especially the air cavities in the skull opening into the nasal passages
squam/ous	(squam- scale) "scalelike"; like, formed of, or covered with scales
sta/sis	(sta- stand) "condition of standing or stoppage"; a stoppage of the flow of some fluid in the body such as blood; reduced peristalsis of the intestines resulting in the retention of feces
strangul/ation	(strangul- a squeezing, choking) "a squeezing or constriction"; inordinate constriction or compression of a tube or a part (as the throat or bowel), especially to a degree that causes a suspension of breathing, circulation, or passage of contents
strict/ure	(strict- compress, draw tight) "compression"; an abnormal narrowing of a passage in the body; stenosis
sym/path/etic	(sym from syn- with + path- disease, feeling) "pertaining to feeling with"; the sympathetic nerve or system of nerves
sym/path/ic/o/	(sym from syn- with + path- feeling, disease + blast- bud + oma- tumor) or

blast/oma

(sympathic- pertaining to the sympathetic nerves + blast- bud, sprout + oma- tumor) "sympathetic cell bud tumor"; a malignant tumor composed of primitive cells which develop into a sympathetic nerve cell

terat/oma

(terat- monster + oma- tumor) "monstrous tumor"; a tumor containing various kinds of embryonic tissue as of hair, teeth, bone, muscle, cartilage

thromb/o/cyt/e

(thromb- clot + cyt- cell) "clotting cell"; a small blood cell that initiates the process of blood clotting; platelet

thromb/osis

(thromb- clot + osis- condition) "clotting condition"; coagulation (clotting) of the blood in the heart or a blood vessel forming a clot

thromb/us

(thromb- clot) "a clot"; the clot attached at the site of the thrombosis

tors/ion

(tors- twist) "a twisting"; the act of turning or twisting; the state of being twisted; the twisting of a body part on its own axis such as a loop of intestine; or the condition of a tooth when it is turned on its long axis

troph/ic

(troph- nourishment, growth) "pertaining to nourishment"; of nutrition; having to do with the processes of nutrition

tum/or

(tum- swell) "a swelling"; a swelling on some part of the body, especially a mass of new tissue growth; neoplasm

tympan/ite/s

(tympan- a drum) "drumlike"; a distension of the abdomen by the accumulation of gas or air in the intestines or abdominal cavity. "Tight as a drum"

xer/o/stom/ia

(xer- dry + stom- mouth) "dry mouth condition"; abnormal dryness of the mouth due to insufficient secretions

Classification of
Operative Procedures

Purpose of this Section

Many of the elements discussed in Medical Terminology are directly concerned with operative procedures. Operative procedures are descriptions of the therapeutic measures that physicians perform for the alleviation or cure of disease and injury. In this section we will discuss the elements used in operative procedures. This discussion will serve to broaden your knowledge of the application of elements as they relate to operations and give you a better appreciation of the meanings of elements as they relate to and differ from each other.

Organization of Operative Procedures

Within body systems and the major organs which are parts of that body system, operative procedures are classified under the following major categories:

> Incision
>
> Excision
>
> Amputation
>
> Introduction
>
> Endoscopy
>
> Repair
>
> Destruction
>
> Suture
>
> Manipulation

Incision   *in/cis/ion*: a "cutting into"; a cut made into a tissue or organ

---

Suffixes and term used to describe types of incisions:
- -/o/tom/y—a "cutting"; the general word ending used to indicate a cutting into a tissue or organ; section
- -cent/esis—a "pricking"; surgical puncture; a needling
- tran/sect/ion—a "cutting across"; a "cross cut"; a long cut; a division by cutting into sections

---

Excision   *ex/cis/ion*: a "cutting out"; surgical removal

The suffix *-ec/tom/y* or "cutting out" is a general word ending used to indicate surgical removal.

Types of excisions:

- ex/cis/ion of les/ion (local ex/cis/ion of les/ion)—surgical removal in which the tissue to be removed (ex/cis/ed) lies within a relatively narrow area; contrast with re/sect/ion
    - les/ion (les- means to hurt or to injure: an injury or other change in an organ resulting in impairment or loss of function.) Tumors, cysts, ulcers are examples of les/ion/s
    - loc/al (pertaining to place) denotes a particular part or specific area of the body; not general; not extensive
- re/section—"cut back"; ex/cis/ion of a considerable portion of an organ or structure; sometimes used to indicate an excision over a wider or deeper area than is implied in a generalized -ec/ tom/y or "excision of lesion"
- radic/al ex/cis/ion—"root cutting out"; going to the "root" or source of a les/ion or other cause; similar to our expression "root out" by which we mean complete removal or eradication
- bi/ops/y—"seeing life"; "viewing life"; the ex/cis/ion of a bit of living tissue from the body for diagnostic examination

Amputation from *am- (amphi-)* "two ways" plus -put/ate "clean, trim, prune"; the surgical cutting off (an arm, leg, etc.)

The term dis/articul/ation—(articul- denotes "joint"; same as *arthr-*) carries the meanings: "joint apart"; the act of surgically disjointing; separation at the joint.

Introduction *intro/duct/ion:* the act of "leading into"; a putting in; insertion

Essentially, intro/duct/ion indicates the insertion or putting of something into the body:

- in/ject/ion—(ject- means "throw"; a tra/ject/ory is the course followed by something thrown; to e/ ject is to throw out); "throw or force in"; the act of forcing or driving (usually a fluid) into some part of the body
- trans/fus/ion—(fus- means "pour," "melt"; to re/fuse is to pour back; give back; put back) "pour across"; the act of pouring across or transferring; specifically, to transfer (blood, blood plasma, saline solution, etc.) into a blood vessel, usually a vein
- im/plant/ation—"plant into"; insertion of a substance, organ, or piece of living tissue into the body
- in/sert/ion—the act of putting or setting something into something else; the act of putting something (usually a device) into the body or body part

    The "something" (devices) may be wires, pins, nails; dentures or other prosthetic devices; orthodontic appliances, pacemakers, etc. or, the device may be briefly introduced such as in:
    - cath/et/er/ization—the insertion of a cath/et/er for the introduction or withdrawal of fluids
    - in/tub/ation—the insertion of a tube, usually for the passage of air or fluids

Endoscopy *end/o/scop/y*: "observe within"; the act of examining visually the inside of a hollow organ of the body

The instrument used for such examination is an endo/scop/e. Endo/scop/es have developed into versatile devices. They are not limited to viewing alone but may also be equipped to obtain biopsies, excise tissue, drain fluids, remove foreign bodies, divide adhesions, insert and inject substances.

Repair to put back in good condition after damage; to restore; renew; set right; remedy

-plasty—the word ending used to generally indicate repair

plast/ic repair of_____ —also used in the same sense of *-plasty* or repair

The element *plas-* means "to form"; "to mold." We have learned that the word ending *-plas/ia* means "forming," "growth," "development." Plast/ic surgery is the branch of surgery concerned with the repair or restoration of lost, injured, or deformed parts of the body, chiefly by the transfer of tissue. Plasma (sometimes shortened to plasm) means "something formed"; used mostly to indicate the fluid portions of the blood.

Plast/ic repair, or *-plasty*, can encompass such surgical procedures on body parts as:
- lengthening
- shortening
- restoration
- reconstruction
- revision

Other repairs are designated as by the following terms and endings:
- graft—transplantation of a piece of skin, bone, or other living tissue from one body, or place on a body, to another
- -stom/y—"making a mouth"; a surgical opening into a specified part or organ frequently for drainage
- -ana/stomy (ana/stom/osis)—"make a mouth again"; interconnection; surgical joining of one hollow or tubular organ with another
- fistul/ization—the surgical creation of an opening into a hollow organ, or of an opening between two structures that were not previously connected
- open reduction—(a re/duct/ion "lead back" is the correction of a fracture or hernia): correction (re/duct/ion) of a fracture after exposing the fracture by an incision
- -pexy—word ending meaning fastening, fixing in place; securing; making fast fixation: the operation of holding, suturing, or fastening in a fixed position
    suspension:—"hang up"; to hang from a support
- -desis—word ending meaning joining or tying
- fus/ion—to bind together; frequently the immobilizing of a joint; arthr/o/desis; artificial ankyl/o/sis. (Ankylosis means a "sticking together" condition, artificial ankylosis means a surgical "sticking together" or fus/ion of a joint, hence, is synonymous with arthr/o/desis.)

- stabilization—to make steady or firm; again, frequently by fusing some of the bones in the joint; arthr/o/desis
- trans/plant/ation: "planting across"; to transfer (tissue or an organ) from one individual, or part of the body, to another; graft

Destruction   the act of obliterating, doing away with de/bride/ment (literally to unbridle); the cutting away of dead or contaminated tissue from a wound to prevent infection

The following suffixes denote various forms:
- -clas/is—"breaking"; the act of breaking

    fracturing—the surgical breaking of a bone to correct a deformity

    re/fracturing—the operation of breaking over again a bone which has been fractured and has united with a deformity

- -tripsy, -trity—word endings indicating the act of crushing

    crushing—applying pressure so as to destroy a structure or substances such as stones (calculi) in the body

- -lysis—word ending indicating loosening, freeing, or division of adhesions (adhesions denote the fibrous tissues that join together body parts which normally are separate; it typically results from inflammation): the removal of adhesions; the surgical severing of the fibers which are abnormally uniting body parts

☞ **Note:** "adhesion" carries the same "sticking together" idea that we use in the word "adhesive."

Stripping is an operative procedure for varicose veins in which large sections of the veins are removed.

Suture   the act or method of joining together the two edges of a wound or incision by stitching or similar means

"Suturing" may be applied in closure of a wound and of a fistula

The word ending -rrhaphy denotes suturing.

The medical term lig/ation means tying off blood vessels or other structures during the performance of an operation.

Manipulation   literally, to operate with the hand or hands; treatment by using the hands

You may be familiar with some conditions that are treated by the skillful manipulation of the physician's hands.

In deliveries at term:
- obstetric delivery
- conversion of position—in case the fetus needs to be turned in the uterus (breech presentation)
- obstetric extraction—in the event the mother needs assistance in expelling the fetus from the uterus
- version—a term to cover a variety of internal and external manipulations to ease or expedite delivery. (remember vers- "turn"?)
- application of or delivery by forceps—the use of a tong-like instrument (forceps) designed to extract the fetus by the head from the birth canal

In dislocations and simple fractures:
- manipulation and appilcation of—plaster, splint, or traction apparatus
- closed reduction—of fractures, that is, fractures that can be corrected with manipulation without the need for incision to expose the fracture
- Removal of—drains, dressings, packing, sutures, wires, etc.

Dilation or stretching:
- -tasia, -tasis—word endings denoting the act of enlarging a passage or hollow organ by stretching

◾ Alphabetical List of Elements ◾

Element	Audionym	Meaning	Lesson	Section/Appendix
a		noun ending, name of thing from a root	4	Word Terminal
ab	Abe	away from, not	11	One of 350 elements taught
abdomin		the abdomen, belly		Familiar Element Appendix
ac		affected by, having, one who is affected by	3	Word Terminal
ac		comparing "pertaining to," "affected by"	3	Word Terminal
ac		pertaining to	1	Word Terminal
acousti	a cue stick	hearing, sound	6	One of 350 elements taught
acro	acrobat	extremeties	3	One of 350 elements taught
acro		farthest ends plus all parts leading to	3	Reading Assignment
acus,acous		sound	6	Reading Assignment
ad		toward, in the direction of	3	Word Terminal
ad		to, toward	3	Reading Assignment
aden	a den	gland	1	One of 350 elements taught
adnexa	annex	ties, connections	7	One of 350 elements taught
adreno	(not required)	adrenal gland	12	One of 350 elements taught
ae		plural ending for words ending in "a"	4	Word Terminal
aer	air (plane)	air	8	One of 350 elements taught
al		pertaining to	1	Word Terminal
alg		pain	2	Reading Assignment
algeo		pain	2	Reading Assignment
algesi		pain, sensitivity to pain	2	Reading Assignment
algia	algae	painful condition, pain	2	One of 350 elements taught
algio		pain	2	Reading Assignment
alveol	owl field	cavity, socket	8	One of 350 elements taught
ambi, ambo	amp, bee	both, around, on both sides (amb, am, an)	13	One of 350 elements taught
ameb	a me	change	10	One of 350 elements taught
amel		enamel		Diseases Appendix
amyl		starch		Diseases Appendix
amphi, ampho	amp, feet	around, on both sides, in two ways	13	One of 350 elements taught
an, a	an "A"	without, not	10	One of 350 elements taught
an, ian		of, belonging to, person associated with	2	Word Terminal
ana, ano		up, back, again, throughout		Familiar Elements Appendix
ance, ancy		state of condition, the act of	7	Word Terminal
angi	angel	vessel, usually blood	1	One of 350 elements taught
angina		a choking, strangling	14	Reading Assignment
angul		angle		Diseases Appendix
aniso		not equal, inequality	7	Reading Assignment
ant		pertaining to, having characteristics of	4	Word Terminal
ante	ant tea	before	11	One of 350 elements taught
anti	ant eye	against	5	One of 350 elements taught
anti		counteracting, preventing, suppressing	5	Reading Assignment
antr	ant tree	cavity, chamber	7	One of 350 elements taught
apo	apple	away from, separation, lack	14	One of 350 elements taught
appendic	(not required)	appendix	12	One of 350 elements taught
ar		pertaining to, having a connection with	2	Word Terminal
arter	(not required)	artery	12	One of 350 elements taught
arthr	art	joint	1	One of 350 elements taught
ary		pertaining to, having a connection with	2	Word Terminal

Element	Audionym	Meaning	Lesson	Section/Appendix
asthenia	his thin knee	weakness	7	One of 350 elements taught
astr	astronaut	star-shaped	7	One of 350 elements taught
ate		perform, put into action, bring about	3	Word Terminal
ation		a process, condition, action	4	Word Terminal
aur	"R"	ear	6	One of 350 elements taught
auto	auto	self	3	One of 350 elements taught
auto		self-caused, occuring within one's body	3	Reading Assignment
basi	(not required)	base	12	One of 350 elements taught
basi		bottom, lowest part, foundation	12	Reading Assignment
benign	bee "9"	mild, not cancerous	4	One of 350 elements taught
benign		favorable for recovery	4	Reading Assignment
bi	(not required)	two, double, both	12	One of 350 elements taught
bili	bill	bile	5	One of 350 elements taught
bin		two, both	12	Reading Assignment
bio, bi		life		Familiar Elements Appendix
blast	blast	bud, shoot, sprout, embryonic cell	14	One of 350 elements taught
blephar	blue fur	eyelid	1	One of 350 elements taught
bol		throw		Diseases Appendix
brachy	brake	short	13	One of 350 elements taught
brady	braid	slow	4	One of 350 elements taught
brevi		short		Familiar Elements Appendix
bronch	(not required)	bronchus	12	One of 350 elements taught
bucco	bucket	cheek	6	One of 350 elements taught
bucco		as landmark	6	Reading Assignment
bul		cattle		Diseases Appendix
burso	purse sew	sac	3	One of 350 elements taught
calc	calculator	heel, stone	9	One of 350 elements taught
calcar		of lime		Diseases Appendix
cantho	can throw	angle at the end of the eyelid	4	One of 350 elements taught
capit, cep	cap	head	13	One of 350 elements taught
carcer		prison		Diseases Appendix
carcin	car sign	cancer	3	One of 350 elements taught
cardi	card	heart	1	One of 350 elements taught
cata, cath	catalog	down, lower, under, complete (also kath)	13	One of 350 elements taught
cau, caus	cough	burn, burning heat, cauter-searing, burning	13	One of 350 elements taught
cauda	cod liver oil	tail	4	One of 350 elements taught
cauda		"the rear end," directional use	4	Reading Assignment
cav, cavit		hollow		Familiar Elements Appendix
cec	seek	blind passage	5	One of 350 elements taught
cele	seal	hernia, tumor, or swelling	4	One of 350 elements taught
celio	ceiling dome	abdomen	4	One of 350 elements taught
celio		any large cavity of the body, esp. abdomen	4	Reading Assignment
centesis	cent	puncture	5	One of 350 elements taught
cephal	sieve fall	head	3	One of 350 elements taught
cerebr	zebra	brain	1	One of 350 elements taught
cervic	serve hic	neck	2	One of 350 elements taught
cess		go		Diseases Appendix
cheil	cow	lip	4	One of 350 elements taught
chein		to pour		Diseases Appendix
cheir, chir	care (package)	hand	9	One of 350 elements taught
chlor		chlorine		Diseases Appendix
chole	coal	bile	2	One of 350 elements taught

Element	Audionym	Meaning	Lesson	Section/Appendix
chole		gall	2	Reading Assignment
chondr	cone door	cartilage	2	One of 350 elements taught
chyl		gastric juice		Diseases Appendix
cilia	ceiling	eyelash	6	One of 350 elements taught
cilia		hairlike projection	6	Reading Assignment
cine	Sen Sen	move, movement	9	One of 350 elements taught
circum		around, about, on all sides		Familiar Element Appendix
clas, clad	class	break, destroy	13	One of 350 elements taught
cle		small, little	2	Word Terminal
clus		to close		Diseases Appendix
coel		hollow	4	Reading Assignment
col	(not required)	colon	12	One of 350 elements taught
colla	cola	glue, gelatin-like	9	One of 350 elements taught
colpo	cold bow	hollow, vagina	6	One of 350 elements taught
com, con		with, together, completely (col, cor)		Familiar Element Appendix
con		together		Diseases Appendix
contin		to hold, contain		Diseases Appendix
contra	contractor	against, counter	4	One of 350 elements taught
contra		"opposite to," "against"	4	Reading Assignment
cor	core	heart	6	One of 350 elements taught
cord, cor		pertaining to the heart	6	Reading Assignment
corne	corn	horny, horn-like	8	One of 350 elements taught
corne		cornea of the eye	8	Reading Assignment
cost	coaster	rib	3	One of 350 elements taught
counter		"against," "opposite to"	4	Reading Assignment
crani	crane	skull	2	One of 350 elements taught
cret		grow		Diseases Appendix
crine	cry'n	to secrete	7	One of 350 elements taught
cryo	cry	cold	11	One of 350 elements taught
cut	cut	skin	9	One of 350 elements taught
cyan	sign	blue	2	One of 350 elements taught
cyst	sister	sac containing fluid, bladder	2	One of 350 elements taught
cyt	sight	cell	4	One of 350 elements taught
dacry	daiquiri	tear	7	One of 350 elements taught
dactyl	duck tail	finger, toe	8	One of 350 elements taught
dendr	den door	tree, branching (as in nervous system)	6	One of 350 elements taught
dent	dentist	teeth	3	One of 350 elements taught
derm		skin	1	Reading Assignment
dermat	doormat	skin	1	One of 350 elements taught
desis	thesis	binding, fixation	3	One of 350 elements taught
di	dye	twice, double, twofold	14	One of 350 elements taught
dia	diet pill	through, across, apart	14	One of 350 elements taught
digit	dig it	finger, toe	9	One of 350 elements taught
dips		thirst		Diseases Appendix
dis	discus	apart, asunder, away, opposite of	14	One of 350 elements taught
dist		far		Familiar Element Appendix
dors	doors	back	9	One of 350 elements taught
dors		back (as landmark), back side	9	Reading Assignment
duct	duck	tube, channel, canal, lead, draw	13	One of 350 elements taught
duodeno	(not required)	duodenum	12	One of 350 elements taught
duplic		double, twofold		Diseases Appendix

Element	Audionym	Meaning	Lesson	Section/Appendix
dura	door	hard	7	One of 350 elements taught
dyn	dinner	pain	3	One of 350 elements taught
dyn, odyn		pain	3	Reading Assignment
dynam	dynamite	power	10	One of 350 elements taught
dys	dice	bad, out of order	9	One of 350 elements taught
dys		out of order, difficult, painful	9	Reading Assignment
e		means of, instrument for	2	Word Terminal
ectasis	egged a sis	expansion	4	One of 350 elements taught
ecto		situated on the outside, outside	11	Reading Assignment
ectomy	exit Tommy	surgical removal of all or part of	1	One of 350 elements taught
edema	a demon	swelling (by fluid)	8	One of 350 elements taught
edema		"edema of...," or as suffix	8	Reading Assignment
EENT		ear, eye, nose, throat (acronym)		Familiar Elements Appendix
em		blood (form of "hem-" within a word)	2	Reading Assignment
em		variation of "en" before "b," "m," or "p"	9	Reading Assignment
embry		early stage of fertilized egg	12	Reading Assignment
eme		vomit, vomiting	4	Reading Assignment
emesis	hey Mrs.	vomiting	4	One of 350 elements taught
en	hen	in	9	One of 350 elements taught
en, em		in, within, inside	9	Reading Assignment
ence		variation of ance - state or condition, act of	8	Word Terminal
encephal	hen sieve fall	brain	6	One of 350 elements taught
end	the end	inside, within	2	One of 350 elements taught
end		inside	2	Reading Assignment
ent		inside, within, inner (alternate form of "end")	2	Reading Assignment
enter	enter (sign)	intestines (usually small)	1	One of 350 elements taught
ependym	a pendulum	wrapping, a covering	8	One of 350 elements taught
ependym		membrane enclosing brain and spinal cord	8	Reading Assignment
epi	a pea	upon, in addition to	3	One of 350 elements taught
erythro	wreath throw	red	4	One of 350 elements taught
es		plural ending similiar to "-s"	5	Word Terminal
esis		condition or process	4	Word Terminal
esis		go, send		Diseases Appendix
eso		inner, inward	12	Reading Assignment
esophag	(not required)	esophagus	12	One of 350 elements taught
esthesia	has the show	sensation, feeling	4	One of 350 elements taught
esthesia		consciousness	4	Reading Assignment
eu	ukulele	good, well, normal, easy	13	One of 350 elements taught
eury, eur	urinal	broad, wide, opposite of narrow	14	One of 350 elements taught
ex	eggs	out, away from	11	One of 350 elements taught
exo		outside, outward, outer	11	Reading Assignment
exterior		more to the outside	11	Reading Assignment
external		outwardly, outward form, appearance	11	Reading Assignment
extra		outside of, beyond	11	Reading Assignment
extro		on the outside, beyond outer (ext. of ex)	11	Reading Assignment
fac, fic, fect	factory	make, do, cause	14	One of 350 elements taught
fac, fici		face, outer surface, form, figure	14	Reading Assignment
fascia	face	sheet, band	7	One of 350 elements taught
fer		carry		Diseases Appendix
fibr		fiber, filament		Familiar Elements Appendix
fiss, fid	fish	split, cleave	13	One of 350 elements taught

Element	Audionym	Meaning	Lesson	Section/Appendix
fistul	fist	pipe, a narrow passage	8	One of 350 elements taught
flacc		flabby		Diseases Appendix
flex, flect		bend, turn		Familiar Elements Appendix
form		same form, shaped like, resembling	3	Word Terminal
furca	fur coat	fork-shaped	8	One of 350 elements taught
fus		melt, join		Diseases Appendix
gangli	gang	swelling, knot-like mass	9	One of 350 elements taught
gangren		a gnawing away, an eating sore		Diseases Appendix
gastr	gas truck	stomach	1	One of 350 elements taught
gemin	gem	twin, double	9	One of 350 elements taught
gen	Genesis	original, production	3	One of 350 elements taught
gen		bring forth, arise in, the source of; producer	3	Reading Assignment
genesis		process or condition leading to production	3	Reading Assignment
genic, genous		producing, originating, giving rise to	3	Reading Assignment
genit		reproduction, the organs of reproduction	3	Reading Assignment
ger, geron	jar	old, old person, old age	13	One of 350 elements taught
geront		old age, old person	13	Reading Assignment
gingiv	gingerbread (man)	gum	1	One of 350 elements taught
gli		glue		Diseases Appendix
glob		ball		Diseases Appendix
glom	glow	ball	11	One of 350 elements taught
glosso	glossy	tongue	3	One of 350 elements taught
glut		glue		Diseases Appendix
glyco, gluco	glide coal	sweet, sugar	8	One of 350 elements taught
grad	graduate	walk, take steps	9	One of 350 elements taught
grad		stage in a process	9	Reading Assignment
gram	graham cracker	record, write	3	One of 350 elements taught
gran	grandma	grain, particle	9	One of 350 elements taught
granul		little grain, little particle		Diseases Appendix
gravid	gravel*	pregnant	8	One of 350 elements taught
gyn, gynec	guide**	female, woman	13	One of 350 elements taught
h		dropping when not initial letter of word	2	Reading Assignment
halit		breath		Diseases Appendix
hallux	hall "x"	great toe	5	One of 350 elements taught
hard		comparisons of dura, scirrh, scler	7	Reading Assignment
helio	heel	sun, light	7	One of 350 elements taught
hem(at)	hem	blood	2	One of 350 elements taught
hemi		part of	2	Reading Assignment
hemi	hemisphere	half	2	One of 350 elements taught
hepat	he pat	liver	1	One of 350 elements taught
hern		intestine, entrails		Diseases Appendix
hesion		a sticking		Diseases Appendix
heter, (eter)	header	other, different from, opposite	13	One of 350 elements taught
hetero		other, different from, opposite	13	Reading Assignment
histo	his toe	tissue	6	One of 350 elements taught
hom, homo	home	same, like, the same as, equal, resembling	13	One of 350 elements taught
homo		man, humankind	13	Reading Assignment
homeo		like, the same as, equal, resembling	13	Reading Assignment
hormone	harmonize	excite or set in motion	10	One of 350 elements taught
hydro	hydrant	water	3	One of 350 elements taught
hyper	high purr	above, more than normal	2	One of 350 elements taught
hyper		excessive, more than normal	2	Reading Assignment

* Previous Edition: gravity
** Previous Edition: gun, ginn

Element	Audionym	Meaning	Lesson	Section/Appendix
hypno	hypnotist	sleep	7	One of 350 elements taught
hypo	hippo	under, beneath, deficient	2	One of 350 elements taught
hypo		less than normal, below in space	2	Reading Assignment
hyster	his stir	uterus, womb	2	One of 350 elements taught
ia		disease, unhealthy state or condition	1	Word Terminal
ian		belonging to or having some relation to	6	Word Terminal
iasis	oasis	condition, formation of, presence of	4	One of 350 elements taught
iasis		disease process, result of disease	4	Reading Assignment
iatr		heal, treat, cure	2	Reading Assignment
ic		pertaining to	1	Word Terminal
ical		pertaining to	1	Word Terminal
ician		of, belonging to, person who	7	Word Terminal
ics		body of facts, knowledge, matters etc.	4	Word Terminal
id		pertaining to, "being"	5	Word Terminal
ide		chemical compound naming	2	Word Terminal
ile	(not required)	ileum	12	One of 350 elements taught
ili	(not required)	ilium	12	One of 350 elements taught
im		not		Familiar Element Appendix
in		organic compound ending	4	Word Terminal
in, il, im, ir		in, within, inward, into; not		Familiar Element Appendix
infer	inn, fur	under, below	13	One of 350 elements taught
infero		below and, on the outside		Familiar Element Appendix
infra	infra red oven	beneath	11	One of 350 elements taught
integument		skin		Reading Assignment
inter	interpreter	between	11	One of 350 elements taught
inter		between, among, in the midst		Familiar Elements Appendix
interior		something that is within, more to the inside		Familiar Elements Appendix
intern		between (variation of inter)		Familiar Element Appendix
internal		existing or situated within something		Familiar Element Appendix
intra	introduce	within	11	One of 350 elements taught
intra		within, during, between layers, underneath	11	Reading Assignment
intro		in, into, inward, within	11	Reading Assignment
ion		action, condition, resulting from action	3	Word Terminal
ior		roughly "more toward"; "comparative," (English -er)	3	Word Terminal
ir		not		Familiar Element Appendix
iris	I race	rainbow (eye membrane)	8	One of 350 elements taught
is		noun ending, add to root to form name	1	Word Terminal
ism		an abnormal condition	6	Word Terminal
iso	I sew	equal	7	One of 350 elements taught
ist		one who practices, does, is concerned with	2	Word Terminal
ite		a part of the body or bodily organ	6	Word Terminal
itic		pertaining to or affected by inflammation	6	Word Terminal
ition		same as -ation, process, action, condition	7	Word Terminal
itis	I test	inflammation	1	One of 350 elements taught
ity		condition, character	8	Word Terminal
ium		noun end, place, region, lining, covering	2	Word Terminal
ive		of, relating to, having nature or quality of	8	Word Terminal
ization		action or process, -ize + -ation	8	Word Terminal
kerat	carrot	horny, horny tissue	8	One of 350 elements taught
kerat		cornea of the eye	8	Reading Assignment
kin, cin		to move	9	Reading Assignment
kine		general relationship to movement	9	Reading Assignment

Element	Audionym	Meaning	Lesson	Section/Appendix
kinet		movable	9	Reading Assignment
labi	lab	lip	9	One of 350 elements taught
lacrim	lake rim	tear	5	One of 350 elements taught
lact	lacquer	milk	5	One of 350 elements taught
lal	lolli (pop)	speech	11	One of 350 elements taught
lapar	lap	abdominal wall	7	One of 350 elements taught
lapar		lower back and sides	7	Reading Assignment
lapse		fall, falling		Diseases Appendix
laryng	(not required)	larynx	12	One of 350 elements taught
lat		wide		Diseases Appendix
later	ladder	side	9	One of 350 elements taught
leio	lei	smooth	6	One of 350 elements taught
lept	leopard	slender, thin, delicate	14	One of 350 elements taught
les		injure, hurt, wound		Diseases Appendix
let		little, small		Diseases Appendix
leuk	Look (magazine)	white	4	One of 350 elements taught
lien	line (clothes)	spleen	11	One of 350 elements taught
lig	(not required)	ligament	12	One of 350 elements taught
lig		tie, bind	12	Reading Assignment
ligat		to bind, tie	12	Reading Assignment
lim		hunger		Diseases Appendix
lingua	language	tongue	4	One of 350 elements taught
lip	lip	fat	2	One of 350 elements taught
lith	lather	stone	2	One of 350 elements taught
lobo	low bow	section	4	One of 350 elements taught
loc		place		Familiar Elements Appendix
lumbo	lumber	loins	11	One of 350 elements taught
ly		in a manner, way, by way of, toward	4	Word Terminal
lymph	limp	watery fluid, major fluid of the body	14	One of 350 elements taught
lysis	license	loosening, destruction, set free	2	One of 350 elements taught
macro	macaroni	large	11	One of 350 elements taught
macul	Mack (truck)	spot (stain)	5	One of 350 elements taught
mal	mall	bad	11	One of 350 elements taught
mal		abnormal, faulty, poor (inadequate, insufficient)	11	Reading Assignment
malacia	my late show (TV)	soft condition	1	One of 350 elements taught
malign	my leg	bad, harmful	7	One of 350 elements taught
mamm	mammal	breast	9	One of 350 elements taught
mani	maniac	madness, mental disturbance	3	One of 350 elements taught
manu		hand	14	Reading Assignment
mast	mast	breast	3	One of 350 elements taught
mat		variation for roots ending in "m"	2	Reading Assignment
maxill	makes hill	upper jawbone	10	One of 350 elements taught
mechano	mechanic	machine	10	One of 350 elements taught
med	meat	middle	14	One of 350 elements taught
medull		marrow, pith		Diseases Appendix
megal	my gal	enlarged	1	One of 350 elements taught
melan	melon	black	4	One of 350 elements taught
mening	manage	membrane	5	One of 350 elements taught
ment	mint	mind	7	One of 350 elements taught
mes		middle, intermediate		Reading Assignment
meta	metal cabinet	beyond, change, transformation, after	14	One of 350 elements taught
metabole	met a bull	change	8	One of 350 elements taught
metr	meter	uterus	10	One of 350 elements taught
mi	mice	less	14	One of 350 elements taught
micr	microphone	small	9	One of 350 elements taught
mio, meio		less, smaller	14	One of 350 elements taught

Element	Audionym	Meaning	Lesson	Section/Appendix
mono		one, alone, single, limited to one part		Familiar Elements Appendix
morph	mower roof	form, shape, finger	14	One of 350 elements taught
motil		movement		Diseases Appendix
motility		movement		Diseases Appendix
multi		many, much, more than one		Familiar Elements Appendix
muscul		muscle		Familiar Elements Appendix
my	my eye	muscle	2	One of 350 elements taught
myco	my comb	fungus	5	One of 350 elements taught
myel	mile	marrow	5	One of 350 elements taught
myring	my ring	eardrum	4	One of 350 elements taught
narc, narcot		numbness, stupor, apathy		Familiar Elements Appendix
nas		nose		Familiar Elements Appendix
necr	neck	dead	14	One of 350 elements taught
neo	kneel	new	10	One of 350 elements taught
nephr	nephew	kidney	1	One of 350 elements taught
ness		state, quality, instance of being	5	Word Terminal
neuro	Nero	nerve or nervous system	10	One of 350 elements taught
nex		join	7	Reading Assignment
nomaly		distributed		Diseases Appendix
non		not		Diseases Appendix
ocul	a kool (drink)	eye	7	One of 350 elements taught
ocul		relationship to the eye, landmark use	7	Reading Assignment
odont	Oh don't	tooth	4	One of 350 elements taught
odyn		pain	3	Reading Assignment
oid	void	like, resembling	2	One of 350 elements taught
olfact	oil factory	smell, odor, to smell	13	One of 350 elements taught
ologist	hollow chest	a specialist in the study of	1	One of 350 elements taught
ology	hollow cheese	study of	1	One of 350 elements taught
oma	Oh Ma	tumor	1	One of 350 elements taught
oma		swelling, mass of new tissue growth	1	Reading Assignment
omat		tumor	2	Reading Assignment
oment	"O" men	covering (of internal abdominal organs)	8	One of 350 elements taught
on		noun ending; name forming from root	6	Word Terminal
onco	uncle	tumor, mass, or swelling	5	One of 350 elements taught
onych	onyx	nail, claw	5	One of 350 elements taught
onych		fingernail, toenail	5	Reading Assignment
oo		egg or ovum	8	Reading Assignment
oophor	over	ovary	8	One of 350 elements taught
opac		dark, shaded		Diseases Appendix
ophthalm	up thumb	eye	2	One of 350 elements taught
opia		suffix denotes condition of vision, sight	2	Reading Assignment
opt		seeing, vision, light, visible, relationship to vision or sight	2	Reading Assignment
or	oar	mouth	5	One of 350 elements taught
or		action, result, performer, functional, functions	3, 8	Word Terminal
orchi	orchid	testis	6	One of 350 elements taught
orchi		male reproductive gland	6	Reading Assignment
orexia		desire, appetite		Diseases Appendix
orth	Orthodox (Church)	straight, correct, normal	13	One of 350 elements taught
osis	Oh sis	condition, any condition	1	One of 350 elements taught
osmo	I smoke	odor	10	One of 350 elements taught
oss		bone	2	Reading Assignment
osse		bone	2	Reading Assignment
ossi		bone	2	Reading Assignment
ost	ostrich	bone	2	One of 350 elements taught

Element	Audionym	Meaning	Lesson	Section/Appendix
oste		bone	2	Reading Assignment
ostomy	Oh stop Tommy	to create an opening	2	One of 350 elements taught
otic, otid		ear as landmark, situated in ear area		Reading Assignment
oto	"O" toe	ear	5	One of 350 elements taught
otomy	Oh Tommy	cut into, incision into	1	One of 350 elements taught
ous		full of, abounding in, having	3	Word Terminal
ov		egg, ovar as egg container	5	Reading Assignment
ovar	over	egg (the female reproductive cell)	5	One of 350 elements taught
ovario	(not required)	ovary	12	One of 350 elements taught
pachy	pack	thick	13	One of 350 elements taught
pact		press		Diseases Appendix
palat		palate, the roof of the mouth		Familiar Elements Appendix
palpebr	pile of people	eyelid	6	One of 350 elements taught
pan	pan	all	10	One of 350 elements taught
pant		variation of pan, all, completely, the whole	10	Reading Assignment
papill		nipple		Diseases Appendix
para	parachute	beside, beyond	2	One of 350 elements taught
para		beyond, wrong, faculty, disordered	2	Reading Assignment
pariet	parrot	wall	8	One of 350 elements taught
part	part	labor, bring forth	7	One of 350 elements taught
part		to separate from	7	Reading Assignment
path	path, (of daisies)	disease	1	One of 350 elements taught
pect, pector	pecked	chest, breast, thorax	14	One of 350 elements taught
ped		foot or child	7	Reading Assignment
pelv		pelvis, ring of bones in hip area	12	Reading Assignment
pelvi	(not reqired)	pelvis	12	One of 350 elements taught
penia	pen	decrease	3	One of 350 elements taught
peps, pept	pepsi	digest	9	One of 350 elements taught
per	purr	throughout, through, thoroughly, excessively	14	One of 350 elements taught
peri	pear	about, around	9	One of 350 elements taught
peri		peri, o, _____ium, peri, o, _____eum, tissue	9	Reading Assignment
peri		surrounding, enclosing, covering	9	Reading Assignment
petechiae		small spots		Diseases Appendix
pexy	pecks egg	suspension, fixation	5	One of 350 elements taught
pexy		surgical act of fastening or securing	5	Reading Assignment
phage	page	to eat	8	One of 350 elements taught
phage		swallowing	8	Reading Assignment
phak	vacuum cleaner	lens	10	One of 350 elements taught
pharmac	farm axe	drug	11	One of 350 elements taught
pharyng	(not required)	pharynx	12	One of 350 elements taught
phleb	flip	vein	6	One of 350 elements taught
phob	foe	fear	9	One of 350 elements taught
phon	phone	voice, sound	6	One of 350 elements taught
phon		speech or body sounds	6	Reading Assignment
phor		carrier	8	Reading Assignment
phot	photo	light	9	One of 350 elements taught
phrag, phrax	fur rag	fence, to fence in, wall off, block up	13	One of 350 elements taught
phren	friend	mind	8	One of 350 elements taught
phren		diaphragm	8	Reading Assignment
physio	physics (book)	nature	6	One of 350 elements taught
physio		the body (as opposed to the mind)	6	Reading Assignment
pica		magpie (omniverous eater)		Diseases Appendix

Element	Audionym	Meaning	Lesson	Section/Appendix
pilo	pile on	hair	6	One of 350 elements taught
plak	plaque	plate	8	One of 350 elements taught
plak		a patch of eruption	8	Reading Assignment
plaque		a patch, a flat area	8	Reading Assignment
plasia	play show	development or growth	6	One of 350 elements taught
plast	plastic (cement)	surgical repair, plastic repair	1	One of 350 elements taught
plast		renewal, reforming reconstruction	1	Reading Assignment
platy	plate	flat, broad	13	One of 350 elements taught
plegia	pledge	paralysis	11	One of 350 elements taught
plegia		loss of power	11	Reading Assignment
pleur	pliers	pleura (membrane), rib, side	9	One of 350 elements taught
pleura		membrane covering the chest cavity	9	Reading Assignment
plexus	plexiglass	braid, an interweaving or network	6	One of 350 elements taught
pne		air or breathing	8	Reading Assignment
pnea		breathing	8	Reading Assignment
pneum	name	lung, air	8	One of 350 elements taught
pneum, pneumat		relationship to air or respiration	8	Reading Assignment
pneumon		relationship to lungs	8	Reading Assignment
pod	pod	foot	7	One of 350 elements taught
poly	polish	much, many	10	One of 350 elements taught
post	post office	after, behind	10	One of 350 elements taught
poster	poster	back part, behind, rear	13	One of 350 elements taught
pre	pray	in front of, before	10	One of 350 elements taught
pro	pro (golfer)	in front of, before	9	One of 350 elements taught
proct	Proctor & Gamble	anus	2	One of 350 elements taught
proct		designating rectum, anal canal	2	Reading Assignment
proli	parolee	offspring	11	One of 350 elements taught
proxim	peroxide	nearest, near	14	One of 350 elements taught
pseud	false teeth	false, imaginary, spurious	13	One of 350 elements taught
psycho	cycle	mind	2	One of 350 elements taught
ptosis	toe sis	falling, drooping	3	One of 350 elements taught
pty		saliva, spittle		Diseases Appendix
ptyal	tile	saliva (pertaining to)	8	One of 350 elements taught
puer	pure (gold)	child	11	One of 350 elements taught
pulmon, pulmo	pull moon	lung	8	One of 350 elements taught
pulmon		lung as landmark	8	Reading Assignment
pyle, pyloro	pie	gate	5	One of 350 elements taught
plyor		"gatekeeper"	5	Reading Assignment
rachi	rake	spinal column	9	One of 350 elements taught
radi	radio	ray	8	One of 350 elements taught
radic	radish	root	8	One of 350 elements taught
ramus	ram	branch	10	One of 350 elements taught
re		back, back again, contrary, opposite		Familiar Elements Appendix
ren	rain	kidney	6	One of 350 elements taught
retro	retreat	backwards	3	One of 350 elements taught
retro		contrary to the usual or natural course	3	Reading Assignment
rhag, rrhag	raging river	burst forth, break, burst, rupture	14	One of 350 elements taught
rhagad		a split, crack, fissure	14	Reading Assignment
rrhagia		heavy bleeding	14	Reading Assignment
rhaphy	raffle	suture, suturing	3	One of 350 elements taught
rhe, rrhe	reed instrument	flow, to flow	14	One of 350 elements taught
rhexis	wrecks	break, burst	3	One of 350 elements taught

Element	Audionym	Meaning	Lesson	Section/Appendix
rhexis		rupture, forcible tearning apart	3	Reading Assignment
rhin	rhinoceros	nose	1	One of 350 elements taught
rrh		rrh vs. rh in elements	3	Reading Assignment
rrhex		to break, burst, rupture	14	Reading Assignment
ruct		belch		Diseases Appendix
rug	rug	wrinkle, fold, crease	6	One of 350 elements taught
rupt		break		Diseases Appendix
sacro	(not required)	sacrum	12	One of 350 elements taught
salpingo	Sally Bingo	tube	6	One of 350 elements taught
salpingo		especially the uterus	6	Reading Assignment
sarc	shark	flesh	11	One of 350 elements taught
schiz	skis	to split, cleave	13	One of 350 elements taught
scirr	skirt	hard	7	One of 350 elements taught
scirrh, scirr		variation of scirr, hard cancerous tumor	7	Reading Assignment
sclera	scholar	hard	7	One of 350 elements taught
scol, scoli	school	curved, twisted, crooked	14	One of 350 elements taught
scolec		worm-shaped	14	Reading Assignment
scop	scope	look, observe	2	One of 350 elements taught
secret		set apart, hidden		Diseases Appendix
sect		a cut or division, to cut or divide		Familiar Elements Appendix
sedat	seated	quiet, calm	8	One of 350 elements taught
semen	seaman	seed	4	One of 350 elements taught
semi	semi colon	half	10	One of 350 elements taught
semi		partially	10	Reading Assignment
sen		old		Diseases Appendix
sept	sipped	wall, fence	7	One of 350 elements taught
sept		dividing wall or membrane	7	Reading Assignment
sin		curve, fold, bend		Diseases Appendix
sinus	sign us	hollow space	7	One of 350 elements taught
skelet		skeleton, the bony framework of the body		Familiar Elements Appendix
somato	sew my toe	body	7	One of 350 elements taught
somni	saw my knee	sleep	11	One of 350 elements taught
spas	space	pull, draw	11	One of 350 elements taught
spasm	spaceman	involuntary contraction	1	One of 350 elements taught
sphenic	sphinx	wedge, wedge-shaped	5	One of 350 elements taught
spiro	sparrow	coil	5	One of 350 elements taught
spiro		winding, twisting	5	Reading Assignment
splanchn	"S" plank	internal organs, viscera	14	One of 350 elements taught
splen	(not required)	spleen	12	One of 350 elements taught
spondyl	spun doll	spinal column or vertebra	4	One of 350 elements taught
squam	squash*	scale	5	One of 350 elements taught
sta, stas, ste	stand	stand, to cause to stand, set, fix	14	One of 350 elements taught
steno	stenographer	narrow, contracted	4	One of 350 elements taught
stenosis		constriction of a passage in the body	4	Reading Assignment
steth		chest	2	Reading Assignment
sthen		strength, strong	7	Reading Assignment
stip		press		Diseases Appendix
stom, stomy		new opening, a mouth or opening	6	Reading Assignment
stoma	stone	mouth or opening	6	One of 350 elements taught
strangul		a squeezing, choking		Diseases Appendix
strept	strap**	twist	3	One of 350 elements taught
strict	strict	draw tight, narrowing	10	One of 350 elements taught

* Previous Edition: squaw
** Previous Edition: strip

Element	Audionym	Meaning	Lesson	Section/Appendix
sub	submarine	under, beneath, below	5	One of 350 elements taught
sub		less than	5	Reading Assignment
super		above, relation to supra	3	Reading Assignment
super		over, above, higher in quantity or quality		Familiar Elements Appendix
supra	soup	above, over	3	One of 350 elements taught
syn, sym	cymbals	together	10	One of 350 elements taught
tarso	tar	ankle region, instep; framework of the eyelid	7, 9	One of 350 elements taught
tas, tend, tens		to stretch	11	Reading Assignment
tegument	tag you men	covering or skin	10	One of 350 elements taught
tein (tan, ten)		to stretch	11	Reading Assignment
tele		distant, far away	2	Reading Assignment
ten		stretch, a stretcher, stretching (extend)	11	Reading Assignment
tens	tents	stretch	11	One of 350 elements taught
terat		monster, monstrous		Diseases Appendix
tetan		stretched, spasm	14	Reading Assignment
thalam	the lamb	inner chamber	6	One of 350 elements taught
thel	the "L"	nipple	11	One of 350 elements taught
therap	(not required)	therapy	12	One of 350 elements taught
therm	thermometer	heat	10	One of 350 elements taught
thorac	throw rock	chest	5	One of 350 elements taught
thromb	trombone	lump, clot	11	One of 350 elements taught
thyro	(not required)	thyroid	12	One of 350 elements taught
tic		pertaining to	4	Word Terminal
ton	ton	stretching, a stretching, tension	14	One of 350 elements taught
top		place, locality, localized	7	Reading Assignment
tope	top	place	7	One of 350 elements taught
tors, tort		twist, turn		Familiar Elements Appendix
tox		poison		Familiar Elements Appendix
trache		windpipe	7	Reading Assignment
trachel	tray coal	neck or neck-like structure	7	One of 350 elements taught
tract		draw		Diseases Appendix
trans	trains	through, across, beyond	4	One of 350 elements taught
trauma		shock, stress, injury	10	Reading Assignment
traumat	laundromat	wound, injury	10	One of 350 elements taught
tres		hole, opening		Diseases Appendix
tri	(not required)	three	12	One of 350 elements taught
tri		involving three, triply, third	12	Reading Assignment
trich	trick	hair	10	One of 350 elements taught
trip	trip	rub, friction	3	One of 350 elements taught
tripsy		crushing	3	Reading Assignment
trophy	trophy	development, growth	3	One of 350 elements taught
trophy		nutrition, nourishment	3	Reading Assignment
trus		thrust, push		Diseases Appendix
tum		swell		Diseases Appendix
tumor	two more	swelling	11	One of 350 elements taught
turbin	turban	shaped like a top	10	One of 350 elements taught
tympan	tin pan	eardrum or its enclosure	6	One of 350 elements taught
ular		pertaining to; pertaining to a small version	2	Word Terminal
ule		small, little	2	Word Terminal
ul		small		Diseases Appendix
ultra		beyond, excessive		Familiar Elements Appendix
um		noun ending, add to root to form name	1	Word Terminal

Element	Audionym	Meaning	Lesson	Section/Appendix
umbilic	a bill lick	navel	6	One of 350 elements taught
ure		result of action, means of action, device	3	Word Terminal
ureter	(not required)	ureter	12	One of 350 elements taught
urethr	(not required)	urethra	12	One of 350 elements taught
us		noun ending, name forming from root	5	Word Terminal
utero	(not required)	uterus	12	One of 350 elements taught
vaso	vase	vessel	4	One of 350 elements taught
vena	(not required)	vein	12	One of 350 elements taught
ventr	vent	front, belly, abdomen, cavity	13	One of 350 elements taught
vermi		worm, worm-like	12	Reading Assignment
vert, vers	vertebrae	turn	13	One of 350 elements taught
vertebr		vertebra, bones of the spinal column		Familiar Elements Appendix
vesic	vest sick	bladder	5	One of 350 elements taught
vestibule	vest bull	entrance	11	One of 350 elements taught
vestibule		space or cavity at entrance to a canal	11	Reading Assignment
viscero	vice row	organ	5	One of 350 elements taught
viscero		internal organ, internal organs	5	Reading Assignment
volv	valve	to roll, turn, roll over, a turning	14	One of 350 elements taught
volut		a turning or rolling motion	14	Reading Assignment
vulse	false	twitch or pull	10	One of 350 elements taught
xer	zero	dry	14	One of 350 elements taught
y		act or result of act, condition, quality	1	Word Terminal

Interpretation Exercise Answers

LESSON 1
1-1. removal, excision / gland
1-2. disease / vessel(s)
1-3. inflammation / joint(s)
1-4. repair / eyelid
1-5. study / heart
1-6. softening / brain
1-7. inflammation / skin
1-8. removal, excision / stomach
1-9. intestines
1-10. stomach / intestines
1-11. inflammation / gum(s)
1-12. study / liver
1-13. inflammation / stomach / intestines
1-14. softening / kidney(s)
1-15. enlargement / liver
1-16. condition / kidney(s)
1-17. study / disease(s)
1-18. study / skin
1-19. tumor / gland
1-20. condition / stomach
1-21. kidney
1-22. disease / brain, cerebrum
1-23. repair / gum(s)
1-24. nose
1-25. contraction / intestine(s)

LESSON 2
2-1. pain / muscle
2-2. inflammation / neck
2-3. removal, excision / gallbladder
2-4. cartilage
2-5. puncture, puncturing / skull
2-6. blue, bluish / skin
2-7. pain / bladder, urinary bladder
2-8. inside, within / heart
2-9. blood
2-10. removal, excision / half, part / liver
2-11. excessive / pain
2-12. deficient, low, under / liver
2-13. removal, excision / uterus
2-14. tumor / muscle / fat
2-15. enlargement / liver
2-16. stone(s)
2-17. tumor / vessel(s) / muscle
2-18. like
2-19. study / eye
2-20. disease / bone / joint
2-21. opening / stomach / intestines
2-22. around / bladder
2-23. repair / anus, rectum
2-24. mind
2-25. observing, viewing

LESSON 3
3-1. blue / extremities
3-2. destruction, disintegration / body, self
3-3. inflammation / sacs, bags, pouches
3-4. cancerous / tumor / gland
3-5. head
3-6. rib(s) / cartilage
3-7. teeth, tooth
3-8. fusing, binding / joint
3-9. outer, surface / skin
3-10. producer / disease

3-11. observation, examination, inspection / tongue
3-12. record, recording / heart
3-13. pouch, bag, sac / water
3-14. obsession / largeness, bigness, greatness
3-15. removal, excision / breast(s)
3-16. pain / extremities
3-17. deficiency, lack / water
3-18. drooping, dropping, falling / eyelid(s)
3-19. behind, in back of / heart
3-20. suture, suturing / muscle
3-21. rupturing, rupture, tearing / uterus
3-22. twisted
3-23. above, over / liver
3-24. crushing / stone
3-25. over, excessive / development

LESSON 4
4-1 mild, non-cancerous
4-2. slow / heart
4-3. corner
4-4. tail
4-5. herniated, hernia / muscle, (muscle hernia)
4-6. incision, cut, abdominal
4-7. cancerous, cancer / tumor / lip
4-8. against, counter
4-9. blood / cell
4-10. stretching, expansion / vessel
4-11. vomiting / bile, gall
4-12. deficiency / red / cells
4-13. study / sensation, feeling
4-14. condition / stones
4-15. white / cell
4-16 tongue
4-17 incision, cutting / lobe, section
4-18. condition / black
4-19 observation, inspection, examination / eardrum, inner ear
4-20. teeth, tooth
4-21. study / semen
4-22. vertebra / spinal column
4-23. condition / narrowing
4-24. through, across / skin
4-25. dilation, relaxation / vessel

LESSON 5
5-1. production
5-2. bile, bile duct(s), (bile, bile duct(s) and gallbladder)
5-3. one
5-4. puncture, puncturing / joint
5-5. big, great / toe
5-6. tears
5-7. milk
5-8. spot, blotch
5-9. inflammation / membrane, membranes
5-10. condition / fungus
5-11. inflammation / bone / bone marrow, marrow
5-12. tumor / breast(s)
5-13. white / nail(s), fingernail(s), toenail(s)
5-14. around, about / mouth

5.15. near / ear
5-16. produced / ovary, ovaries
5-17. fixation, fastening / uterus
5-18. removal, excision / stomach / opening
5-19. wedge
5-20. resembling, like / coil
5-21. scaly, platelike
5-22 below, beneath / tongue
5-23. chest / abdomen
5-24. bladder
5-25. organ(s)

LESSON 6
6-1. hearing
6-2. ear / skull, cranium
6-3. above, over / cheek
6-4. eyelashes, eyelash
6-5. inflammation / vagina
6-6. heart
6-7. like, resembling / branch
6-8. inflammation / brain
6-9. tissue / cell
6-10. tumor / smooth / muscle
6-11. fixing / testicle
6-12. eyelid(s)
6-13 narrowing, constricting / vein(s)
6-14. recording, record / heart
6-15. study / body
6-16. cyst / hair
6-17. development, growth / breast
6-18. below, beneath / network, tangle, braid
6-19. above, over / kidney(s)
6-20. wrinkles, folds, creases
6-21. opening / tube
6-22. pain / mouth
6-23. inner / chamber
6-24 eardrum
6-25. navel, belly button

LESSON 7
7-1. join, joined, joined to
7-2. sinus, cavity, hollow space, hollow
7-3. weakness / eye(s)
7-4. tumor / star / cells
7-5. excessive, above normal, high, over / secretion
7-6. production, creation / tears
7-7 hard
7-8. sheet, band
7-9. sensitivity / sun, sunlight
7-10. study / sleep
7-11. same, equal, like
7-12. opening / stomach / abdominal
7-13. cancerous, bad, harmful
7-14. mental, mind
7-15. disease / eye(s)
7-16. before / labor, birth
7-17. foot, feet
7-18. hard / breast(s)
7-19. condition / hardening, hardness
7-20. wall, partition
7-21. hollow space, cavity
7-22. bodily / disease, disorder
7-23. ankle
7-24. fixed, localized, "place of" / pain
7-25. inflammation / muscle(s) / neck

LESSON 8
8-1.   air
8-2.   pit, cavity
8-3.   horn-like, horny
8-4.   examination / finger
8-5.   swelling / fingers / toes
8-6.   membrane, covering
8-7.   passage
8-8.   fork
8-9.   increase, high / sugar
8-10.   pregnant
8-11.   colored, rainbow
8-12.   horny
8-13.   transformation, change
8-14.   covering
8-15.   ovary
8-16.   walls, wall
8-17.   pain / swallowing
8-18.   slowness / mental, mind
8-19.   white / plates
8-20.   inflammation / lungs, lung
8-21.   saliva
8-22.   kidneys / lungs
8-23.   x-rays, rays
8-24.   root, lowermost part
8-25.   calms, quiets

LESSON 9
9-1.   stone
9-2.   inflammation / joints / hand(s)
9-3.   motion, moving
9-4.   glue, gelatin-
9-5.   skin
9-6.   finger / toe
9-7.   back / side, sides
9-8.   difficult, labored, bad / swallowing, eating
9-9.   in / head
9-10.   mass, knotlike mass, swelling, tumor
9-11.   pairs, twos, twins, doubles
9-12.   walking / toes
9-13   particle
9-14.   lips / teeth
9-15.   side
9-16.   record, recording / breast
9-17.   small / heart
9-18.   slow / digestion
9-19.   inflammation / around / gland
9-20.   fear
9-21.   light
9-22.   membrane
9-23.   front / brain
9-24.   puncture, puncturing / spinal column
9-25.   framework, edge, tarsus

LESSON 10
10-1.   changing
10-2.   lack / blood, red blood cells
10-3.   muscular, muscle / force, power, strength
10-4.   deficiency
10-5.   upper / jawbone
10-6.   machines
10-7.   blood / uterus
10-8.   new / disease
10-9.   a nerve, the nerves
10-10. smell, odors
10-11. removal, excision / whole, total / uterus
10-12. inflammation / lens, crystalline lens
10-13. much, excessive, many / sound, sounds

10-14. behind, after / mouth
10-15. front, front part / cranium, skull
10-16. branch
10-17. somewhat, partially, half / malignant, bad, cancerous
10-18. drawing tight, tightening, narrowing
10-19. binding together, fusion, togetherness
10-20. covering / skin
10-21. high / heat, temperature
10-22. injury, wound
10-23. white, whiteness, whitening / hair
10-24. top
10-25. twitching, pulling, contraction, contractions

LESSON 11
11-1.   away / from
11-2.   before / labor, birth
11-3.   cold / blooded
11-4.   produced / outside
11-5.   small / rounded, round, (ball-shaped)
11-6.   below, beneath / mammary
11-7.   between / muscles
11-8.   within, inside / spinal, vertebral
11-9.   disease, disorder / speech
11-10. spleen
11-11. loins
11-12. large, big / eye, eyes
11-13. bad, faulty
11-14. study / light / drugs
11-15. (all) total / paralysis
11-16. (children) off spring
11-17. childhood, childish, children
11-18. fleshy, flesh
11-19. disease/ sleep, sleeping
11-20. muscle / spasms, contractions
11-21. stretches, tenses
11-22. nipple
11-23. clotting, clot / cell
11-24. swelling, mass
11-25. entrance

LESSON 12
12-1.   disease / adrenal
12-2.   removal, cutting out, excision / appendix
12-3.   hardening / arteries
12-4.   base
12-5.   both, two / feet
12-6.   inflammation / bronchial
12-7.   colon / perforated, punctured
12-8.   opening / gall bladder / duodenum
12-9.   falling down, dropping, prolapse, downward displacement / esophagus
12-10. ileum
12-11. ilium
12-12. larynx / study / neck
12-13. connects, ties, holds
12-14. rupture, breaking apart / ovary
12-15. incising, cutting, cutting into / pelvis
12-16. pain / pharynx
12-17. sacrum
12-18. enlargement / spleen / liver
12-19. physical
12-20. excessive, high / thyroid
12-21. three / testicles
12-22. ureter / urine
12-23. condition / narrowing / urethra
12-24. inflammation / uterus
12-25. vein

LESSON 13
13-1.   both
13-2.   feet / both, two
13-3.   short, shortness of / lip
13-4.   head / foot
13-5.   down
13-6.   burning / pain
13-7.   breaking / bone
13-8.   tube, channel, passage
13-9.   normal, good / blood
13-10. splitting
13-11. old, aged / extremities
13-12. resembling, like / female, woman
13-13. opposite
13-14. same
13-15. below, under / side
13-16. smell, smelling
13-17. correcting, straightening / teeth
13-18. thick / skin, skinned
13-19. blocking, fencing / urethra
13-20. flat / feet
13-21. behind / above
13-22. false, imaginary / pregnancy
13-23. split / mind
13-24. front, belly side, abdominal region
13-25. twist, turn

LESSON 14
14-1.   lack / produce, reproduce
14-2.   little / bud
14-3.   double, two / uteruses
14-4.   loosening / apart
14-5.   cut / apart, across
14-6.   wide, broad / head
14-7.   face
14-8.   slender, thin, skinny / fingers / toes
14-9.   lymph / gland, node
14-10. middle / nose
14-11. development, developing / change, changes
14-12. bone / lessening, disintegration, reduction
14-13. single, same / shape, form, figure
14-14. excision, removal, cutting away / dead
14-15. pain / chest
14-16. through / skin
14-17. nearest, nearer, closest, closer
14-18. intestinal / bleeding
14-19. flow / through
14-20. condition / curvature, crookedness
14-21. pain / internal organ
14-22. stop, check, curtail, fix / blood
14-23. tension, pressure
14-24. rolled, twisted, coiled, turned, folded / together
14-25. dry / skin

Element Recognition Answers

Lesson 1

gastr/o/hepat/itis	hepat/o/nephr/o/megal/y
aden/o/path/y	blephar/o/plast/y
cardi/o/megal/y	rhin/ologist
enter/o/plast/y	gingiv/ectomy
dermat/ologist	arthr/itis
path/osis	enter/o/gastr/itis
cerebr/o/malacia	path/ology
angi/o/path/ology	dermat/oma
nephr/ologist	cardi/o/malacia
hepat/itis	aden/otomy
arthr/ectomy	arthr/o/plast/y
blephar/o/spasm	angi/ology
rhin/ology	blephar/otomy
gingiv/osis	gastr/itis
angi/o/megal/y	path/ologist
nephr/o/malacia	aden/ectomy
hepat/oma	gingiv/itis
cerebr/o/path/y	nephr/otomy
gastr/ectomy	cerebr/itis
enter/o/megal/y	rhin/o/path/y
cardi/ology	dermat/itis

Lesson 2

gastr/algia	lith/o/cyst/otomy
crani/o/cerebr/al	ophthalm/o/my/otomy
end/o/chondr/al	proct/o/scop/y
hemi/crani/osis	nephr/algia
lip/oid	crani/otomy
hyper/chol/ia	end/angi/itis
cyst/o/lith/ectomy	hyper/aden/osis
chole/lith	cyst/ectomy
hypo/hem/ia	chole/cyst/itis
hyster/o/scop/y	hypo/lip/osis
cyst/ostomy	rhin/o/scop/y
para/proct/itis	hyster/o/lysis
angi/o/lysis	para/hepat/ic
cervic/o/plast/y	chondr/o/lysis
chondr/o/dermat/itis	cervic/itis
cyan/osis	hemat/oma
hemat/ologist	oste/o/lip/o/chondr/oma
oste/o/arthr/o/path/y	lip/o/arthr/itis
psych/o/path/ology*	lith/o/scop/e*
lip/o/chondr/oma	ophthalm/o/my/itis
my/oid	proct/o/spasm

*Also psycho/path/ology   *Also lith/o/scope

Lesson 3

cost/o/chondr/al	epi/cyst/itis
chole/cyst/o/gram	hydro/hepat/osis
acro/path/ology	angi/o/gram
angi/o/rrhexis	acro/megal/y
carcin/o/gen/esis	cardi/o/rrhexis
hydro/penia	carcin/oma
path/o/gen	hypo/gen/esis
burso/lith	burso/path/y
retro/cervic/al	retro/cardi/ac
lith/o/tripsy*	cephal/o/path/y
arthr/o/desis	aut/ology
glosso/plast/y	epi/derm/is
auto/trophy	hydr/ology
supra/cerebr/al	mani/a
blephar/o/ptosis	gloss/algia
my/odyn/ia**	troph/ology
mast/aden/itis	supra/cost/al
glosso/rrhaphy	gastr/o/ptosis
dent/oid	cervic/odyn/ia**
cephal/o/gen/esis	mast/o/carcin/oma
auto/cyst/o/plast/y	my/o/rrhaphy

*Also lith/o/trip/sy or lith/o/trips/y

**Also my/o/dyn/ia   **Also cervic/o/dyn/ia

Lesson 4

lob/otomy	lingu/al
emet/ology	spondyl/odyn/ia*
contra/ception	leuk/o/derm/a
odont/iasis	cantho/rrhaphy
trans/derm/ic	cheil/itis
brady/gloss/ia	cyst/o/cele
angi/ectasis	celi/oma
cyt/o/path/ology	erythro/penia
odont/o/trip/sis	vas/algia
leuk/o/cyt/o/penia	melan/o/derm/a
hyper/esthesia	myring/o/plast/y
cantho/lysis	spondyl/o/lysis
steno/cephal/y	lob/ectomy
cheil/o/plast/y	lith/iasis
enter/o/cele	trans/fusion
semen/ologist	brady/cardi/a
celi/algia	cardi/ectasis
erythro/cyan/osis	cyt/o/gen/esis
vaso/rrhaphy	odont/o/ptosis
melan/o/carcin/oma	cheil/otomy
caud/al	myring/o/scop/e*

*Also spondyl/o/dyn/ia   *Also myring/o/scope

Lesson 5

ov/i/gen/esis
thora/centesis
oto/lith/iasis
bili/ous
squam/ous
mening/o/cerebr/itis
cec/o/pexy
macul/a
nephr/o/pexy
onc/osis
or/alogy
sub/cost/al**
myel/o/malacia
spir/oid
lacrim/otomy
viscero/ptosis
lact/i/gen/ous
onych/o/malacia
thorac/o/my/odyn/ia*
pyloro/sten/osis
vesic/o/cele

myel/o/mening/itis
anti/myco/tic
myco/myring/itis
onc/ology
sub/gloss/itis
viscer/algia
lact/o/cele
onych/o/rrhexis
thorac/o/scop/y
myc/osis
anti/plast/ic
hepat/o/pexy
cec/um
sphen/oid/otomy
vesic/otomy
ov/oid
arthr/o/centesis
ot/odyn/ia*
bili/gen/esis
meninge/o/rrhaphy
sphen/o/cephal/y

*Also thorac/o/my/o/dyn/ia   *Also ot/o/dyn/ia
**Previous Edition: subcutaneous (sub/cutan/eous)

Lesson 6

physio/lysis
bucco/gingiv/al
palpebr/itis
colpo/hyper/plasia
aur/i/scop/e*
acoust/ic
colpo/celio/centesis
phon/o/cardi/o/gram
leio/my/oma
ren/o/troph/ic
orchid/o/ptosis
encephal/o/malacia
cili/o/gen/esis
dendr/oid
phleb/o/lith/iasis
pil/osis
hist/oid
stomat/o/plast/y
tympan/ectomy
salping/ostomy
leio/derm/ia

ren/i/cardi/ac
orchi/o/myel/oma
encephal/o/lith
cili/ectomy
phleb/o/rrhexis
pil/ology
histo/lysis
stomat/o/malacia
tympan/otomy
umbil/ectomy
salpingo/cele
physi/ology
bucco/lingu/al
palpebr/al
hypo/plas/ia
colpo/ectasis
phon/o/path/y
stomat/algia
salping/itis
hist/oma
colpo/rrhaphy

*Also aur/i/scope

Lesson 7

helio/path/ia
astr/o/cyt/oma
lei/asthenia
fasci/o/desis
iso/gen/esis
tarso/megal/y
top/algia
pod/arthr/itis
malign/ant
adnex/o/gen/esis
ocul/o/path/y
lapar/o/chole/cyst/otomy
dacry/o/cyst/o/rhin/o/sten/osis
scler/aden/itis
somat/asthenia
trachel/odyn/ia*
sinus/otomy
hypno/gen/ic
scirrh/o/blephar/onc/us
antr/ostomy
end/o/crin/o/path/y

adnex/ectomy
lapar/o/salping/otomy
dacry/o/aden/algia
scler/o/sten/osis
somat/esthesia
trachel/o/my/itis
sinus/itis
hypn/algia
antr/ectomy
crin/o/gen/ic
heli/osis
astr/o/cyt/e
gastr/asthenia
fasci/o/rrhaphy
iso/cyt/osis
tarso/ptosis
top/esthesia
pod/odyn/ia*
dacry/o/lith/iasis
somato/psych/ic
sinus/oid

*Also trachel/o/dyn/ia   *Also pod/o/dyn/ia

Lesson 8

pneum/o/melan/osis
phag/o/cyt/o/lysis
phren/asthenia
irid/ectasis
kerat/o/gen/esis
pulmon/itis
ptyal/o/lith/iasis
alveol/odont/al
oophor/o/hyster/ectomy
oment/o/rrhaphy
sedat/ive
furc/al
radi/ectomy
radi/o/carcin/o/gen/esis
fistul/ectomy
cephal/edema
dactyl/o/spasm
metab/ology
pariet/itis
ependym/itis
gravid/o/cardi/ac

aer/enter/ectas/ia
hyper/glyco/derm/ia
alveol/algia
oment/itis
radic/al
dactyl/o/gram
metabol/ism
ependym/o/cyte
aer/end/o/card/ia
glyco/penia
pneum/o/hypo/derm/a
phag/o/mani/a
phren/itis
irid/o/ptosis
kerat/o/derm/a
pulmon/ectomy
ptyal/o/gen/ic
phren/o/path/y
kerat/oma
ptyal/o/lith/otomy
ependym/a

Lesson 9

tarso/cheil/o/plast/y	pleur/algia
cheir/o/pod/algia	mamm/ectomy
calcul/o/gen/esis	rachi/otomy
cine/plast/y	top/o/phob/ia
dors/algia	phot/esthes/is
grad/uated	dys/chol/ia
granul/o/cyt/o/penia	cut/itis
labi/o/myc/osis	en/cephal/algia
micr/o/angi/o/path/y	peri/cerebr/al
pept/o/gen/ic	pro/gloss/is
mamm/o/plasia	tars/itis
later/al	cheir/arthr/itis
rachi/o/dynia*	calcan/e/odyn/ia
phag/o/phob/ia	cines/algia
phot/o/dermat/osis	gran/ul/o/cyte
dys/oste/o/gen/esis	labi/ology
sub/cutan/eous	micr/o/lith/iasis
en/cephal/o/mening/o/path/y	pleur/o/chole/cyst/itis
mamm/o/plast/y	dys/end/o/crin/ia
peri/gloss/itis	en/cyst/ed
pro/ptosis	peri/oste/oma

*Also rachi/o/dyn/ia

Lesson 10

dynam/o/gen/esis	ameb/a
osm/esthesia	neo/phob/ia
traumat/o/path/y	therm/algesi/a*
trich/o/troph/y	syn/chil/ia
maxill/ectomy	metr/o/colpo/cele
an/esthesia	pan/cyt/o/lysis
phac/o/scler/osis	poly/path/ia
pre/tympan/ic	neuro/ot/ology
strict/ur/otomy	dynam/o/scop/y
turbin/ectomy	osmo/phob/ia
ameb/oid	traumat/ologist
neo/phren/ia	trich/o/rrhexis
hormon/o/gen/esis	maxill/itis
therm/o/hyper/esthesia	an/algesi/a**
syn/dactyl/ism	phac/o/malacia
post/cardi/otomy	pre/cost/al
metr/o/phleb/itis	therm/o/lysis
pan/hemat/o/penia	syn/oste/ology
poly/trich/ia	metr/o/sten/osis
neuro/troph/asthenia	poly/cheir/ia
turbin/otomy	neuro/traum/a

*Also therm/alges/ia
**Also an/alges/ia

Lesson 11

thromb/o/cyst	sarco/myc/es
ab/lact/ation	macro/esthesia
phren/o/plegia	lal/o/plegia
thele/plast/y	intra/osse/ous
ex/enter/itis	inter/chondr/al
tumor/i/gen/esis	infra/psych/ic
vestibul/otomy	cry/algesi/a*
sarc/aden/oma	glom/oid
proli/fic	somni/fic
macr/onych/ia	pharmac/o/mani/a
lal/o/neur/osis	lumb/odyn/ia**
intra/leuk/o/cyt/e	thromb/o/gen/esis
inter/palpebr/al	a/blephar/ia
infra/cost/al	para/plegia
cry/esthesia	thel/algia
mal/practice	ex/odont/ia
glom/angi/oma	lien/o/cele
hyper/tens/ion	infra/maxill/ary
somni/path/y	lumbo/dors/al
pharmac/o/dynam/ics	lien/o/ren/al
lumbo/cost/al	lal/o/phob/ia

*Also cry/alges/ia
**Also lumb/o/dyn/ia

Lesson 12

arteri/o/scler/osis	ile/o/ile/ostomy
appendic/o/lith/iasis	ili/o/cost/al
thyro/a/plasia	therm/o/therap/y
splen/o/cele	sacro/lumb/ar
ovario/rrhexis	pharyng/o/cele
adreno/megal/y	ureter/o/sten/osis
basi/crani/al	laryng/o/rhin/ology
pelv/o/spondyl/itis	basi/later/al
ven/ectas/ia	pelv/i/therm*
urethr/o/cyst/itis	urethr/o/rrhaphy
utero/plast/y	utero/lith
sacr/arthr/o/gen/ic	bronch/o/phon/y
pharyng/o/plegia	esophag/o/myc/osis
duodeno/chole/doch/otomy	tri/cheir/ia
ureter/o/nephr/ectomy	ile/o/col/otomy
laryng/o/centesis	cryo/therap/y
bronch/o/pneum/o/path/y	ili/o/lumb/ar
col/ostomy	arteri/o/strep/sis
esophag/o/col/o/gastr/ostomy	thyro/ptosis
bi/ram/ous	splen/o/myel/o/malacia
tri/dactyl/ism	ovari/o/salping/ectomy

*Also pelvi/therm

Lesson 13	**Lesson 14**
ambi/later/al	apo/gen/y
amphi/carcin/o/gen/ic	blast/oma
brachy/cephal/ic	di/morph/ic
capit/ate	dia/meter
cata/plas/ia*	dis/able
dia/clas/ia	eury/cephal/ous
duct/al	lept/o/derm/ic
eu/esthesia	lymph/aden/oma
sub/fiss/ure	med/ial
ger/o/derm/a	meta/morph/osis
gyn/o/path/y	mi/o/card/ia*
heter/odont	mono/morph/ous
hom/odont	necr/ectomy
infer/ior	pect/us
olfact/ology	per/nas/al
orth/odont/ics	proxim/al
pachy/derm	hem/o/rrhag/e
dia/phrag/m	dia/rrhe/a
platy/pod/ia	scoli/osis
poster/ior	splanchn/odyn/ia**
pseud/o/esthesia	hem/o/sta/sis
schiz/o/phren/ia	ton/ic
ventr/al	volv/ul/us
in/vert	xer/o/cheil/ia

*Also cata/plasia

*Also mio/cardi/a   **Also splanchn/o/dyn/ia

MEDICAL TERMINOLOGY 350

100% Award
Final Test

Name_____ Date_____

Number Correct:	_____
Possible Score:	_____ 350 _____
Percent Correct:	_____ %

☞ **Important**:

Clearly print the meaning of each element in the blank where indicated. A space has been provided for you to also include its audionym as an aid in recalling the meaning. This step is optional. You will be scored on the meanings of the elements only.

	Element	Audionym	Meaning
1.	gastr-		
2.	cardi-		
3.	megal-		
4.	-itis		
5.	dermat-		
6.	plast-		
7.	cerebr-		
8.	path-		
9.	-ectomy		
10.	enter-		
11.	-osis		
12.	-otomy		
13.	aden-		
14.	angi-		
15.	-oma		
16.	nephr-		
17.	hepat-		
18.	arthr-		
19.	blephar-		
20.	-ologist		
21.	rhin-		
22.	gingiv-		
23.	-malacia		
24.	-ology		
25.	spasm		

Element	Audionym	Meaning
26. -algia		
27. crani-		
28. end-		
29. hemi-		
30. -oid		
31. hyper-		
32. cyst-		
33. chole-		
34. hypo-		
35. -scop-		
36. hyster-		
37. -ostomy		
38. para-		
39. -lysis		
40. cervic-		
41. chondr-		
42. cyan-		
43. hem(at)-		
44. ost-		
45. psycho-		
46. lip-		
47. my-		
48. lith-		
49. ophthalm-		
50. proct-		

Name _____

Element	Audionym	Meaning
51. cost-		
52. -gram		
53. acro-		
54. rhexis		
55. carcin-		
56. -penia		
57. gen-		
58. burso-		
59. retr(o)-		
60. trip-		
61. strept-		
62. -desis		
63. mani-		
64. glosso-		
65. -trophy		
66. supra-		
67. -ptosis		
68. -dyn-		
69. mast-		
70. -rrhaphy		
71. dent-		
72. cephal-		
73. auto-		
74. epi-		
75. hydro-		

Element	Audionym	Meaning
76. lobo-		
77. -emesis		
78. contra-		
79. -iasis		
80. trans-		
81. brady-		
82. -ectasis		
83. cyt-		
84. odont-		
85. leuk-		
86. -esthesia		
87. cantho-		
88. steno-		
89. cheil-		
90. -cele		
91. benign		
92. semen		
93. celio-		
94. erythro-		
95. vaso-		
96. melan-		
97. cauda-		
98. lingua-		
99. myring-		
100. spondyl-		

Name _____

Element	Audionym	Meaning
101. ovar-		
102. -centesis		
103. oto-		
104. bili-		
105. squam-		
106. mening-		
107. cec-		
108. macul-		
109. -pexy		
110. onco-		
111. or-		
112. sub-		
113. spiro-		
114. lacrim-		
115. viscero-		
116. lact-		
117. onych-		
118. thorac-		
119. pyle-		
120. vesic-		
121. sphenic-		
122. myel-		
123. anti-		
124. myco-		
125. hallux-		

Element	Audionym	Meaning
126. physio-		
127. bucco-		
128. palpebr-		
129. -plasia		
130. rug-		
131. aur-		
132. acousti-		
133. colpo-		
134. phon-		
135. leio-		
136. cor		
137. ren-		
138. orchi-		
139. encephal-		
140. thalam-		
141. plexus		
142. cilia		
143. dendr-		
144. phleb-		
145. pilo-		
146. histo-		
147. stoma-		
148. tympan-		
149. umbilic-		
150. salpingo-		

Name _____

Element	Audionym	Meaning
151. helio-		
152. astr-		
153. -asthenia		
154. fascia		
155. iso-		
156. tarso-		
157. -tope		
158. pod-		
159. malign-		
160. adnexa-		
161. ocul-		
162. lapar-		
163. dacry-		
164. ment-		
165. part-		
166. scler(a)-		
167. somato-		
168. trachel-		
169. sinus		
170. hypno-		
171. sept-		
172. scirr(h)-		
173. antr-		
174. -crine		
175. dura		

Element	Audionym	Meaning
176. pneum-		
177. phage		
178. phren-		
179. corne-		
180. plak-		
181. iris		
182. kerat-		
183. pulmon-		
184. ptyal-		
185. alveol-		
186. oophor-		
187. oment-		
188. sedat-		
189. furca-		
190. radic-		
191. radi-		
192. fistul-		
193. edema		
194. dactyl-		
195. metabol(e)-		
196. pariet-		
197. ependym-		
198. gravid		
199. aer-		
200. glyco-		

Name _____

Element	Audionym	Meaning
201. tarso-		
202. cheir-		
203. calc-		
204. cine-		
205. digit		
206. dors-		
207. gangli-		
208. gemin-		
209. grad-		
210. gran-		
211. labi-		
212. micr-		
213. peps-		
214. pleur-		
215. mamm-		
216. colla-		
217. later-		
218. rachi-		
219. phob-		
220. phot-		
221. dys-		
222. cut-		
223. en-		
224. peri-		
225 pro-		

Element	Audionym	Meaning
226. mechano-		
227. dynam-		
228. osmo-		
229. traumat-		
230. trich-		
231. maxill-		
232. an-, a-		
233. phak-		
234. pre-		
235. strict-		
236. turbin-		
237. ameb-		
238. semi-		
239. neo-		
240. hormone		
241. therm-		
242. syn-, sym-		
243. vuls-		
244. post		
245. metr-		
246. tegument		
247. pan-		
248. poly-		
249. ramus		
250. neuro-		

Name _____

Element	Audionym	Meaning
251. thromb-		
252. ab-		
253. -plegia		
254. ante-		
255. thel-		
256. ex-		
257. lien-		
258. tumor		
259. vestibule		
260. puer-		
261. sarc-		
262. proli-		
263. macro-		
264. lal-		
265. intra-		
266. inter-		
267. infra-		
268. cryo-		
269. mal-		
270. glom-		
271. tens-		
272. spas-		
273. somni-		
274. pharmac-		
275. lumbo-		

Element	Audionym	Meaning
276. arter-		
277. appendic-		
278. thyro-		
279. splen-		
280. ovario-		
281. adreno-		
282. basi-		
283. pelvi-		
284. vena-		
285. urethr-		
286. utero-		
287. sacro-		
288. pharyng-		
289. duodeno-		
290. ureter-		
291. laryng-		
292. bronch-		
293. col-		
294. esophag-		
295. bi-		
296. tri-		
297. ile-		
298. ili-		
299. lig-		
300. therap-		

Name _____

Element	Audionym	Meaning
301. ventr-		
302. vert-		
303. eu-		
304. ambi-		
305. amphi-		
306. brachy-		
307. capit-		
308. cau-		
309. clas-		
310. duct-		
311. fiss-		
312. ger-		
313. heter-		
314. infer-		
315. hom-		
316. olfact-		
317. orth-		
318. gyn-		
319. pachy-		
320. phrag-		
321. poster-		
322. cata-		
323. platy-		
324. pseud-		
325. schiz-		

Element	Audionym	Meaning
326. proxim-		
327. scol-		
328. apo-		
329. di-		
330. dia-		
331. eury-		
332. pect-		
333. necr-		
334. mi-		
335. morph-		
336. dis-		
337. fac-		
338. lept-		
339. lymph-		
340. meta-		
341. -rrhag		
342. sta-		
343. ton-		
344. volv-		
345. splanchn-		
346. -rrhe		
347. med-		
348. xer-		
349. per-		
350. blast-		

Name _____

A Message from the Author

Congratulations for having successfully completed this course. You have now joined the more than two million individuals who, with our Total Retention System™, have mastered the basic design of medical terminology and achieved the ability and skill to interpret over 11,000 medical terms.

Be sure to use this Learning Guide to periodically review the application of the system along with the 350 elements, their audionyms and meanings. This will assure your continued retention and ability to easily interpret medical terms. Over time as you become more familiar with the elements, your need for the system will diminish.

I trust you have enjoyed our Total Retention System™ and that it has made learning medical terminology a pleasurable experience for you.

Dean Vaughn
www.deanvaughn.com

DCM/INSTRUCTIONAL SYSTEMS, a division of DCM Systems Incorporated *is the exclusive publisher and supplier of the Dean Vaughn Total Retention System™ Instructional Series for Allied Health.*